How to Quit Drinking Without AA
A Complete Self-Help Guide

Revised 2nd Edition

Jerry Dorsman

THREE RIVERS PRESS
NEW YORK

Published by Three Rivers Press, New York, New York.
Member of the Crown Publishing Group, a division of Random House, Inc.
www.crownpublishing.com

THREE RIVERS PRESS and the Tugboat design are registered trademarks of Random House, Inc.

Originally published by Prima Publishing, Roseville, California, in 1997.

How to Quit Drinking Without AA was originally published by New Dawn Publishing Company, 551 Elk Mills Road, Box 71, Elk Mills, MD 21920.

Chapter 2: The Johns Hopkins Medical Institution's Test for Alcoholism. By permission.

Chapter 14: Zig Ziglar's Seven Steps to Achieving Goals from *Goals,* copyright 1986, Zig Ziglar. By permission Nightingale-Conant Corporation (1-800-525-9000).

Printed in the United States of America

Library of Congress Cataloging-in-Publication Data
Dorsman, Jerry.
How to quit drinking without AA / Jerry Dorsman. —Rev. 2nd ed.
      p. cm.
Includes bibliographical references and index.
1. Alcoholics—Rehabilitation. 2. Self-help techniques. 3. Alcoholics Anonymous.
I. Title.
HV5278.D58 1994
362.29'28—dc20   93-23555
                                                                               CIP

ISBN 0-7615-1290-X

20 19 18 17 16

Second Edition

To every alcoholic drinker who chooses
to make a change . . . this book is dedicated
to your success.

CONTENTS

Preface   xiii
Introduction: How This Book Can Help   1

PART ONE: What Does Alcohol Mean to You?   7

1 A New View of Alcoholism   9
A Way of Coping   10
Something You Learned   12
Just a Part of You   14
Your Own Special Struggle   16
A Physical Addiction   18
A Disease Controlled by Diet   30

2 Are You an Alcoholic Drinker?   37
You're the Best Judge   38
  Test #1: One Question   38
Stop Hiding   39
    Worksheet #1: Denials and Excuses   41
Now Take Another Look   48
    *Test #2: The Johns Hopkins Medical
        Institution's Test for Alcoholism   48*
What's the Verdict?   50

3 Are the Benefits Worth the Problems?   51
The Benefits of Drinking   52
    *Worksheet #2: My Reasons
        for Drinking   53*
Problems Caused by Drinking   57
    Practice #1: Dialogue with Body   59
    *Checklist #1: Checklist of Medical
        Problems   62*

Will You Need Inpatient Care?   69
Your Evaluation of the Problems   70
   Worksheet #3: Problems You'd Like
    to Avoid   70
Do You Want to Quit?   74
   Worksheet #4: Reasons for Quitting   75

PART TWO: Planning Your Own Personal Approach
        to Quitting   79

4   What About AA?   81
How AA Can Help   82
   Practice #2: Try a Few Meetings   84
Drawbacks to AA   84
It's Your Choice   89
   Worksheet #5: My Decision about AA   89

5   How to Break a Habit   91
All About Habits   92
Breaking Habits, Making Changes   96
   Practice #3: Pick a Few Habits and
    Break Them   102
What Else Can You Do?   105
   Checklist #2: Alternatives to Drinking   106
Yes, You Can Change   112

6   Healing Through Diet   114
The Importance of Diet   115
A Matter of Balance   116
Recommended Foods and Beverages   121
Healthful Ways of Cooking and Eating   140
To Supplement or Not to Supplement   146
How to Make the Change   152
How to Handle Cravings   161
   Practice #4: Start Your New Diet   165

7 Building Inner Strength   166
Exercise   168
   Worksheet #6: Plan Your Own
      Exercise Program   169
   Practice #5: Begin Doing It   175
Relaxation Techniques   175
   Checklist #3: Relaxers: What Works Best
      for You?   181
Assertiveness Training   181
   Practice #6: Assertive Responses: How to
      Remain Centered   183
Stress Management and Coping
   Techniques   185
   Checklist #4: 22 Surefire Stress
      Reducers   185
Friendship   189
   Practice #7: Find One Good Friend   190

8 Thirty Additional Ways to Renew
   Yourself   192
The Amazing Success of Acupuncture   193
Massage . . . for Health and Relaxation   195
Biofeedback   196
Bodywork/Body Movement   197
Hypnosis   198
Autogenic Training/Self-Hypnosis   199
Visualization   199
Affirmations   201
Subliminal Suggestion   202
A Clinic or a Live-In Program   204
Solitude and Self-Reflection   211
Healing with Laughter   211
Turn Off Your TV   212
Fasting   214
Intestinal Cleansing   216
Herbal Remedies   217

Aromatherapy   219
Homeopathy   220
Chiropractic   220
A Chemical Deterrent to Drinking   221
*Alternative Approaches to Quitting
    Drinking   222*
Counseling/Psychotherapy   229
Group Therapy   230
Light Therapy   231
Expressive Arts Therapy   232
Hug a Friend   233
Religion   234
Spiritual Healing   236
Charity/Altruism   239
Growing in Love   240
     *Worksheet #7: Which Techniques Will
        You Do?   241*

**PART THREE: Quitting and Making It Work
          for You   245**

 9 Okay—Pick a Day   247
    Use Everything You've Learned So Far   248
       Worksheet #8: Your Master Plan   248
    Promise Someone   249
    Make a Contract   250
       *Worksheet #9: Contract to Quit
           Drinking   250*
    Pick a Day and Quit   251
       Worksheet #10: Your Day   253

10 Getting a Successful Start   254
    Coping with Urges   255
       *Worksheet #11: 169 Ways to Cope
           with Urges   256*

How Close Can You Get to Alcohol?   256
   *Practice #8: Avoiding Drinking
      Situations*   257
For Anyone Who Asks You . . .   259
   Checklist #5: Why I'm Not Drinking   260

11 **Fifteen Common Problems and How
to Solve Them**   264
Anxiety   265
Depression   265
Anger   266
Disturbed Sleep   267
Guilt   267
Overeating   268
Gastrointestinal Distress   269
Visions, Hallucinations   270
Fuzzy Thinking   271
The Same Old Family Situation   271
Sex   272
Friends   273
Setbacks   273
Slips   274
Celebrations   275

12 **Enjoying the Benefits of Not Drinking**   276
Two Big Benefits   276
   *Worksheet #12: How Much Time Do
      You Save?*   277
   *Worksheet #13: How Much Money Do
      You Save?*   279
You Deserve a Reward   280
   Checklist #6: Claim Your Prizes   281
Having Fun   283
   *Worksheet #14: The Benefits
      of Not Drinking*   284

13 Inspirations to Help Make Quitting
Easier   287
Do One Thing at a Time   287
All Things Come to Those Who Wait   289
Old Endings Are New Beginnings   289
Everything Changes   290
Don't Take Anything Too Seriously   290
Live this Very Moment   291
You Can't Have Everything All at Once   292
Hear the Truth Within   292
Your Life Is as Long as You Want It to Be   293
You Can Have this Day for Free   293

14 Making Your Life a Success   295
What Are Your Important Goals?   296
    Worksheet #15: Personal Life Goals   296
*Getting What You Want and Getting Good
    Results Without Alcohol   298*

15 Freedom   300
Feeling Free   301
Steering Clear of Trouble   302
    *Practice #9: Three Ways to Keep
        Your Freedom   303*
A New You   303

Afterword   305
Bibliography and Recommended Reading   307
Index   315
About the Author   321

Acknowledgments

My special thanks . . .

. . . To Charles Bufe for his suggested changes and editorial advice on the revised edition.

. . . To Bob Davis for his editorial advice on the first edition and for his support through the entire project.

. . . To Ken Wiggins for his marketing advice and ongoing friendship.

. . . To Hope Siena, whose given name recalls precisely what she helped me find within myself.

. . . To Kathy Cunningham, whose loving companionship has helped me to claim an ever greater vigor with life.

. . . And to my father, who quit his own alcoholic drinking, but who could have used some other positive ways to renew his health. Long after his death, his brilliance and strength touch me more now than ever before.

Preface

How to Quit Drinking Without AA will help you get sober—and stay that way. With this complete self-help guide, you'll make your own decisions and plan your own successful approach.

The book brings together my 25 years of research, study, and personal experience. It's my life work, and now I offer it to you with confidence. I'm certain you will find on these pages the strongest available program for quitting drinking.

First you'll get some specialized information about alcoholism—the facts you need to know. Then you'll discover the newest techniques for treating the problems alcohol causes.

Armed with the facts and the techniques for curing yourself, you can make a change. You can watch yourself begin to grow. Ready-to-use checklists, worksheets, and practices will help you every step of the way.

You have a chance to renew yourself. By reading this book and following its methods, you can make a major change—a change that will last the rest of your life. When you choose to quit drinking with these methods, you will boost your everyday vitality, find greater happiness, and add many wholesome years to your life.

Soon each day becomes a new beginning. The time to start is now.

Introduction: How This Book Can Help

If you ask people how to quit drinking, most often you'll hear, "Go to AA." Yet among those who need the help, hardly anyone wants to go.

For more than 50 years, Alcoholics Anonymous has been the most recommended approach to quitting drinking. But only 5% of Americans with serious drinking problems belong to AA. Furthermore, among those who join, less than 12% remain in the program for more than three years. These numbers have been established over and over by numerous studies, including AA's own triennial surveys of its membership.

So let's face it. AA misses the vast majority of alcoholics. It simply doesn't work for about 95% of those who need the help.

You may be one of them. For your own reasons, you may have already decided AA is not for you. In that case, you will surely welcome a new approach to cure yourself of alcoholism.

Clearly an alternative is needed, now more than ever. In spite of AA, alcoholism has reached epidemic proportions. Recent statistics show that 19 to 20 million Americans have serious drinking problems, including 5 million teenagers. And the numbers continue to rise.

THE ALCOHOLISM EPIDEMIC

There are about 100 million adult drinkers and 50 million nondrinkers in the United States. If you're a drinking adult, chances are better than one in ten you're an alcoholic drinker.

Among teenagers the odds are worse. About three in ten have serious problems with alcohol. Moreover, the average age for starting drinking keeps dropping. Kids 10 to 14 are now drinking, and many of them become addicted at this young age. Two decades ago, the average starting age was 14 to 18.

In recent years, about 100,000 Americans per year have been dying from alcohol-related causes. Alcoholic drinking increases the risk of death from heart disease, cirrhosis, cancer, mental disorder, immune deficiency diseases (including AIDS), and scores of other physiological problems. In addition, alcohol is implicated in half the driving fatalities, up to 70% of drowning deaths, and about 30% of all suicides. Also, studies among convicted criminals show that heavy drinking contributes to nearly a third of the nation's burglaries, rapes, and assaults.

Currently, the average cost of alcoholism runs an estimated $117 billion annually. This includes medical bills, time lost from work, decreased job efficiency, support for families, and property damage.

But here's the deepest tragedy: Alcoholism causes

turmoil and disruption among family members and leaves emotional scars that can last a lifetime. Uncontrolled drinking is involved in about 40% of family court cases, 25% to 50% of violence between spouses, and about 30% of child molestation cases. A 1987 poll showed that one in four families has a problem with alcohol in the home. Alarmingly, this rate has doubled since 1974.

WHY AA MAY NOT BE THE BEST APPROACH

Quitting drinking can be difficult even under the best circumstances. Without the right approach, it can be nearly impossible. The right approach means *right for you*.

Each person needs to find his or her own way. That means the best program for you will be the one that feels the most comfortable and offers techniques suited to your individual needs. But it's up to you to learn what works for you. You must decide.

Many alcoholic drinkers who plan to quit don't like AA's approach for one reason or another. You may feel this way too. Here are the two main reasons people give for disliking AA:

1. AA offers moral support based on a specific religious philosophy. If the philosophy doesn't match your own, you're more likely to fail, no matter how hard you try. Part of this approach requires a moralistic attitude that many people aren't willing to adopt.

2. AA offers group therapy with a social support network. This can be very successful for those who feel comfortable in groups. Unfortu-

nately, many alcoholic drinkers feel terribly anxious in a group. These people can't function in a group unless they can drink.

There's one other problem with AA. As a major organization, it has been stubbornly resistant to change and has remained basically the same since its inception in 1935. Even when new discoveries have shown how recovering alcoholics can improve their health, AA has not incorporated these techniques into its program. In fact, AA neglects to offer any information on how to treat the physical damage caused by alcoholism.

But such treatment is an essential goal of overall recovery, especially when you consider that alcoholism is a serious metabolic disorder harming every cell of the body. This cellular damage leads to numerous diseases with serious physical and mental side effects. When you quit drinking, you can help yourself immensely by using healing techniques to repair this damage.

The other important treatment goals include the fulfillment of your social, emotional, and spiritual needs. You must have a variety of options. That way, you can choose which options suit your nature and your emotional and moral inclinations. For you, the philosophical premise of AA may be too restrictive.

A NEW SELF-HELP APPROACH

At present, many new alternative programs offer a complete approach to solving the problem of alcoholism. More important, these new programs show much greater success than AA. Three-year cure rates for the new alternatives vary from 50% to 90%, as contrasted with the 12% cure rate of AA.

Many of the new alternatives, including the self-help approach in this book, allow you to choose your own specific techniques. Within a given framework you find what works for you, then begin to use it. In this way, you plan a program uniquely suited to your needs.

The self-help approach in this book is based on one simple premise: *You can take responsibility for your own health*. By doing so, not only will you want to quit drinking, you will learn how. Once you know the specific problems you need to overcome and the best methods to achieve your goals, you can do so with relative ease.

With this book you will:

- examine your individual need for alcohol.
- decide whether you want to quit drinking.
- develop your own treatment plan.
- choose the best techniques that will work for you.
- create your own success.

It's entirely up to you. This self-help approach offers you everything you need: the latest facts, the best new treatment methods, and an organized plan to guide you. Now, more than ever before, you can choose to help yourself.

PART ONE

What Does Alcohol Mean to You?

CHAPTER 1

A New View of Alcoholism

"A moment's insight is sometimes worth a life's experience."
— *Oliver Wendell Holmes, Sr.*

"Knowledge is power."
— *Francis Bacon*

The more you know about a problem, the better equipped you are to resolve it. In this chapter, you'll learn more about alcoholism—why you crave alcohol and what it gives you in return.

Alcoholism changes everything about you. It becomes a way of life, a deeply ingrained pattern with physical, emotional, and even spiritual edges. There are many parts to it.

With the new perspective on alcoholism presented in this chapter, you will take a look at drinking from a drinker's point of view. This will help you get acquainted with the drinker—and the non-drinker—inside you. Then, when you're ready to quit, you can become the nondrinker without any fear of alcohol.

This six-part perspective shows how alcohol affects the whole person. As you read it, you'll gain a complete understanding of alcoholism. Not only will you look at the benefits you gain from alcohol, but you'll also examine the problems it causes.

A WAY OF COPING

Alcohol helps us cope. Our drinking makes us feel better or helps us avoid some problem. Basically, we drink to gain some desired effect. There are hundreds of ways alcohol seems to help. Each person has his or her own unique set of reasons for drinking.

Sometimes we find a different reason for each drink we take. Here's an example: Allen knows he gets nervous around others. Because he's going to a party tonight, he has a couple of drinks. He does this to "calm himself down" and "get ready to meet people." When he gets to the party he still feels uptight, so he has another drink to "loosen up." A couple more drinks help him to "laugh and joke with others." His wife is coming on to him, so he has a couple more drinks to "get in the mood." The last drink at the party is "one more for the road." Back home and before going to bed with his wife, he has another drink to be "a lusty lover." And if he gets through sex without passing out, he has one last drink to "help him sleep."

Alcohol helps Allen cope with these and many more experiences. Alcohol does so much, it's easy to see why people become so devoted to drinking.

Here are a few specific ways alcohol helps. It can help you:

- take risks
- calm yourself down

- overcome shyness
- escape loneliness
- forget some sadness
- feel bolder
- solve problems or forget problems
- overcome depression
- fit into social situations
- remove worry
- suppress anger or get your anger out
- cope with personal stress
- reduce feelings of guilt or shame
- celebrate happy occasions
- ease tensions
- get rid of aches and pains

With so many good effects of drinking, why would anyone want to quit? There are two main reasons: (1) If you continue to drink excessively, alcohol soon stops helping you and actually begins to hurt you, causing more problems for you than it helps you to solve; (2) Most of us, sooner or later, realize we'd rather do something on our own instead of depending on a drug to help us do it.

Early in our drinking careers we're amazed at how easily we can fit alcohol into our lives. But it gets harder and harder. Instead of using alcohol to help now and then, we begin depending on it to help us constantly. We can't get along without it. We stop wanting a drink and start needing a drink.

This is a crucial change. It indicates addiction.

Here's another way to see it. After a while, we start using alcohol to cope with problems that only alcohol is causing. We need a drink to stop the shakes. Or to blot out the memory of our drunken behavior the day before. Or to cut the pain of a hangover. That's how powerful this drug can be. We use it as a medication for so many of our problems—even the problems it itself causes. No wonder we feel we need it!

In Chapter 3, you'll list specific ways alcohol helps you. Then in Chapters 4 through 15, you'll discover many different ways of coping—ways that, in the long run, will work better for you than alcohol ever did.

SOMETHING YOU LEARNED

Alcohol is not an easy drug. It doesn't come with instructions; you have to learn how to use it. In fact, the more you drink, the more there is to learn.

Some of this learning can be fun. When we first start drinking, we learn the many ways alcohol helps us. We think it's great. Then we begin a long process of learning how to gain the most benefits every time we drink. But that means we also spend a lot of time learning to minimize the many problems alcohol can cause.

For instance, I learned early on that alcohol helped me with shyness. It helped so much I quickly began to drink in all social situations. I practiced drinking just enough to get the right buzz for every occasion. I worked on it long and hard. I had to learn how to pace myself so I wouldn't get too drunk too soon and blow my cool.

Learning not to overdrink, to get the perfect glow every time, is difficult. You have to learn your limits. If you drink too much too fast, you might become sick or cause an embarrassing scene. You might get in a bad mood or just downright sloppy. You might get in trouble with the law. Or you might lose control and hurt someone you really care about.

How can you control your drinking all the time? It's hard. In fact, it's almost impossible. There are just too many variables. For instance, whether you get drunk and how fast you get drunk depend on:

- how much you've eaten, what you've eaten, and when
- what your mood was before you started drinking
- how long since your previous drink
- how long since your previous drunk
- how many other toxins your liver is struggling with (such as food preservatives and chemical additives, environmental toxins from the air or water, any drugs you have taken including pre-scription drugs, how much sugar you've consumed and so on).
- how you're consuming your alcohol (how fast, what strength, from what source—beer, wine, or liquor, and even what type of beer, wine, or liquor)
- other variables such as time of month (for women especially, but men also have monthly biological cycles), outside stress factors in your life, whether your body is fighting an illness (even something as simple as a sore throat)

That's a lot to learn. But as alcoholic drinkers, we attempt to learn it all. Our purpose? To gain control over alcohol—so we can get as high as we want, without overdoing it. Some of us become so adept that we can control the variables most of the time.

But when you get this good, surprisingly, there's not much excitement anymore. You normally follow the same routine every day. You maintain a steady alcoholic equilibrium, and after a while it gets boring.

Most alcoholic drinkers lose control of their intake. Not all the time, but often. In some ways it's more exciting to lose control now and then, but it's also dangerous. When we get too drunk, accidents can happen. Serious accidents. So we try to control the uncontrollable and minimize the danger of hurting ourselves and others. As we drink we think, "I can control it if I try." And we keep trying. And trying . . .

JUST A PART OF YOU

Jud would tell anyone sitting next to him at the bar, "I'm an alcoholic . . . there's no two ways about it." Then he'd quaff another brew.

Actually, there *are* two ways about it. A part of you remains nonalcoholic, no matter how much you drink.

This is very important. Why? Because most people label themselves one thing or another, as alcoholic or not alcoholic, but not something in between. Then they act as if they're stuck in their description and have no choice.

Even if you're a down-and-out alcoholic drinker who stays drunk constantly, only a part of you can be considered "alcoholic." Even though all your cells contain alcohol as a result of your alcoholic blood, even though each cell craves alcohol as soon as the alcohol level goes down, each one still retains some integrity. This integrity is provided by alternatives to alcohol: the food you eat, the water you drink, the air you breathe. To be sure, a definite part of you does not depend on alcohol. In fact, this part dislikes alcohol

intensely and fights against it. This part works to pre-
serve your body's natural health.

Donna's friends and relatives could easily see both
sides of her. They would say, "She's okay . . . especially when she's not drinking." Or: "I know deep
down in her heart she's a good person . . . if only she
wouldn't drink so much."

Look closely inside yourself and you'll see two op-
posing forces. One of them is alcoholic. The other is
not.

The part of you that's not alcoholic lies just below
the surface, close at hand. But, as you might expect,
the drunker you are, the harder it is to get in touch
with this part. Still, it's there and it's very strong.
This nonalcoholic part of you has quite a bit of character. It's an interesting side of yourself that you probably don't know too well. The alcohol keeps it hidden.

Yet it's this non-alcoholic part of you that thinks
you might be "alcoholic." It's there the morning after,
shuddering and shaking at what you did to yourself
the night before. The nonalcoholic part of you knows
you have a problem.

It's the *alcoholic part* of you that thinks you're
fine. This part keeps excusing your alcoholic behavior
and hiding your problems from you. This part will do
virtually anything to keep you drinking.

It's the *nonalcoholic* part that sees the problems
alcohol is causing. This part wants to quit drinking.
This is the part of you that has decided to read this
book. It is this part you need to get to know.

Why? Because the nonalcoholic part of you will
win your battle against alcohol. This whole side of
you begins to grow as soon as you quit drinking. Best
of all, this side will help you live a longer, healthier,

and more fulfilling life than you can ever experience by living through your alcoholic side.

YOUR OWN SPECIAL STRUGGLE

"Some of us might find happiness if we would quit struggling so desperately for it."
—William Feather

Part of you is trying to attain happiness through alcohol, but alcoholic drinking involves you in a struggle—one part of you going one way, one part another. You fight with yourself. And you fight with alcohol to get what you want.

The reason? Alcohol helps you but it hurts you too. Your thrills tonight become high blood pressure, headache, nausea, and regrets tomorrow.

So drinking is a challenge. And challenges are fun, right? Alcohol challenges you to get the benefits it brings while finding ways to avoid the problems. Hey, it's not easy!

You try not to get too drunk here, not to make a fool of yourself there. It's a full-time job. You work hard at it. You juggle your schedule to fit as much alcohol into your life as possible. You find novel ways to handle hangovers. This becomes a monumental struggle as hangovers get worse and worse. If you're responsible for earning money, you make an extra effort to get to work on time. You try not to drink on the job, or else try not to drink too much. Sometimes you feel completely helpless. Often you endure a lot of pain.

You'd think if alcohol causes such distress, it

would be easier to quit. And indeed it would be, but for the fact that most of us get completely involved with the struggle itself, so much so that it becomes our own personal life-struggle, the inner story of our lives. And of course we grow to like it.

Here are some reasons we get attached to the alcoholic struggle:

- It's a challenge.
- It gives us a sense of involvement.
- It's like a game—we play hard and try to win.
- Like the concept "no pain no gain," sometimes we need to feel as if we're suffering before we can have a good time.
- It gives us something to complain about.
- It requires strength to keep it up, so it shows how tough we are.
- It's like an adventure—every time we drink we don't know where it will lead.

You may like the alcoholic struggle for any one, or for all, of these reasons. Most of us get involved in our struggles for many different reasons and we may even have different reasons on different days.

"You gotta be tough," my uncle used to say, as he handed my father a drink. Then he'd insist, "Here . . . drink up . . . it builds character."

He was serious, in a joking sort of way. And it's true. Alcohol does build character, but not the kind of character he was talking about. The "alcoholic character" deals with a deeper life-struggle than most people can handle. It's an intense struggle, requiring a great deal of energy.

You feel it every day. You live hard. You go for all

the gusto you can get. And even though you look beat most of the time, and even though you feel exhausted, you continue.

But slowly, over time, you begin to lose it, no matter how tough you are. Granted, you may continue fighting on the surface, but alcohol keeps hurting you inside. Sometimes it feels as if you're fighting for your very life. And, deep down, this is actually what's happening.

Alcohol begins destroying your organs faster than your body can repair them. It speeds the disease process in your body and you begin to have more and more serious illnesses. In a way, it's as if you're deliberately reminding yourself of death, so the life you feel is a true exhilaration.

This requires strength to keep it up. But ultimately you must surrender. You must surrender by giving your life to alcohol, or you must surrender by quitting it altogether.

If you choose to quit, you will find something else to challenge you, something else to give you a sense of involvement; something to work on, spend your time on; something more interesting to struggle with. This book will help you. Here, you'll discover many exciting, workable alternatives—alternatives that will be more fun, bring more rewards, and allow you to be a greater success in your life.

A PHYSICAL ADDICTION

Alcohol could be a free ticket through life if it weren't for the physical addiction. The physical addiction drags you down. You begin drinking more but enjoying it less.

What happens? You go from wanting a drink to

needing a drink. Alcohol becomes your medicine. It seems to cure everything. The problem is, you begin feeling healthy only when you're drinking, and you feel sick whenever you stop.

For Gloria, quitting wasn't easy. Every time she stayed off alcohol for more than a day, she grew nervous and upset, and she began getting angry at everyone around her. Like clockwork, every time, by the end of the day she would say, "I can't stand it anymore! I gotta have a drink." Her drinking no longer seemed a choice.

Gloria could go without alcohol for about a day. Others can go for three or four days or even a week, before they can't stand it anymore and have to have a drink. Other drinkers, especially everyday drinkers, cannot go for more than a few hours. Many of them wake in the middle of the night, needing a drink just to get back to sleep.

Two Signs

There are two signs of the physical addiction. (1) You begin needing more and more alcohol to get the same effects. This is called *increasing tolerance*. (2) You begin to feel that you can't get along without alcohol. You feel more and more pain whenever you try to quit. This sign of addiction is called the *withdrawal syndrome*.

"Tolerance" describes how much alcohol your body can handle. As your body adjusts to alcohol, your tolerance increases. What two drinks did in the beginning may take five, ten, twenty, or even more drinks as tolerance increases. Your body finds its limit. Then, after many years of heavy drinking, tolerance begins to reverse: Cells start breaking down and simply can't handle as much alcohol.

The second sign of physical addiction appears only when you take alcohol away. Your body complains out loud, your nervous system flashes urgent signals to the mind: "Give me another drink to calm me down."

The agitation in the cells can be so great that your whole body can go into convulsions. This is serious. About 20% to 25% die during these convulsions if they don't have medical treatment.

As a rule of thumb, the longer and harder you've been drinking, the more problems you'll experience during withdrawal. The shorter and less excessive your drinking career, the more likely your withdrawal syndrome will look like a hypoglycemic attack. You'll feel fatigued, jumpy, restless, headachy, quick to anger, depressed. Further, these symptoms will disappear temporarily if you eat or drink something sweet, or if you drink alcohol.

Two Causes

Medical research shows two major causes of physical addiction: (1) Your cells adapt to alcohol; and (2) Your body has a problem with alcohol metabolism.

Adaptation in the cells. To your cells, alcohol becomes a way of life. Your blood bathes every cell in alcohol on a fairly regular schedule. Your cells adjust. They grow to expect these doses on time.

Your cells learn to cope with alcohol by defending themselves against its toxic effects. Cell walls harden to retain stability and reduce toxic damage. But as your cells toughen against alcohol, gradually more and more alcohol can be consumed. Your tolerance increases.

In the long run, however, cell walls break down.

At this point, your cells lose their ability not only to keep toxins out but to retain the essential nutrients you get from food. Many of them stop functioning altogether, or start functioning abnormally. That's when your organs (heart, brain, liver), which are nothing more than whole systems of cells, begin to fail.

Your cells show signs of physical addiction another way. They crave alcohol as a food. Alcohol converts almost instantly to glucose in the blood. Your body uses this substance, also known as blood sugar, as food for all the cells. When you drink alcohol, as when you eat a candy bar or drink a soda, the cells get a quick burst of energy. This energy, as you may know, is measured in calories.

Alcoholic beverages pack a lot of calories. Five to ten drinks provide the same amount of calories as a well-balanced meal. But the meal, of course, would have provided essential vitamins, minerals, proteins (amino acids), fats, fiber, and the complex carbohydrates—all of which the body needs to stay healthy. Unfortunately, the simple carbohydrates of alcohol satisfy hunger too well. So when you drink a lot, you usually don't feel like eating a meal, balanced or not.

Your cells adapt yet another way. They grow to crave alcohol for the sedation. Alcohol sedates all your cells. Also, secondary compounds called isoquinolines form in the brain, where they cause heroinlike sedation of the brain and nervous system. That's why, among all the cells, nerve cells react most violently whenever alcohol is taken away. You'll see anything from shaking hands and nervous irritability to convulsive seizures.

Problem with alcohol metabolism. Physical addiction, the body's normal reaction to too much alcohol too often, doesn't affect everyone the same way. A

select group of people, who have a problem metaboliz-
ing alcohol, are especially susceptible.

Alcohol metabolism is normally a simple chemical process. Basically the liver detoxifies the body of
alcohol by breaking alcohol into acetaldehyde (another toxic chemical), and then reducing acetaldehyde
to acetate or acetic acid, which quickly converts to
glucose in the blood. In "alcoholic" drinkers the liver
functions poorly during this second step. It converts
acetaldehyde to acetate at about half the speed of a
"normal" drinker's liver.

This malfunction causes two main problems. First
of all, acetaldehyde builds in the blood. As a powerful
toxin, acetaldehyde adds to the toxic damage alcohol
causes the cells, which start to fight as much to protect themselves from acetaldehyde as from alcohol.

Secondly, acetaldehyde interacts with brain enzymes, creating isoquinolines, those opiatelike chemicals that tranquilize the brain and nervous system.
This chemical byproduct doubles or even triples the
sedative effect of the alcohol. What's more, this added
sedative in the brain dramatically increases the addictive power of alcohol. Because of it, withdrawal becomes more extreme. You go all the way from euphoric sedation while drinking to a high-pitched
buzzing anxiety when you withdraw. How do you get
rid of the anxiety? Alcohol. Or other sedative drugs.

So the metabolic problem causes greater agitation
in your cells, as they're forced to fight another toxin.
But it causes greater sedation as well. That's why,
when you get the alcohol "really working," you're rar-
ing to go yet calm and cool. How can you beat this
high?

And all this because of a glitch in metabolism.
Clearly this glitch is the main reason for your physi-

cal addiction. About 10% of all drinkers have this problem. They are the ones who become "alcoholic."

So why do some livers develop this metabolic problem, while others do not? Why do some livers set the stage for alcoholism by processing alcohol at a slower rate? There are at least five ways the metabolic problem can begin:

- genetic inheritance
- fetal alcohol addiction
- sugar addiction
- overeating
- prolonged excessive drinking

Let's look at each of these in turn.

Genetic inheritance. The "alcoholic metabolism" can be inherited. If your mother or father or any of your four grandparents had a problem with alcohol, you stand a better than average chance of having a problem with it.

What's the average chance? In America, about 10% of all drinkers become alcoholic drinkers. If you have a history of alcoholism in your family, and if you become a drinker, your chances of becoming an alcoholic drinker are anywhere from two to five times greater than average. Instead of a 10% chance, you have a 20% to 50% chance of becoming an alcoholic.

The chance increases because you inherit certain elements of your biochemistry through your genes. Your ability to metabolize alcohol is more likely to be weak if it was weak in one or more of your parents or grandparents. One other point: You may also inherit a weak sugar metabolism, and this can lead to a problem with alcohol metabolism once you start drinking.

So your genetic history plays an important role in the development of alcoholism. If alcoholism runs in your family and if you start drinking, there is a greater than average risk that you will become an alcoholic.

However, you can't say whether you will for sure, based on genetic factors. Even with a strong genetic history of alcoholism, you still have a 50% to 80% chance of not being affected. Obviously, other factors are involved.

Fetal alcohol addiction. A baby can be born with a full-blown alcohol addiction. At birth, the child's liver can have a problem with alcohol metabolism, and he or she can have built up a tolerance to alcohol, exhibit a withdrawal syndrome, and show all the physiological traits that accompany alcoholism.

This can happen to any baby whose mother drank heavily during pregnancy. Why? Because alcohol goes from the mother's blood directly into the fetus: It crosses the placenta. What's worse, if the mother has the alcoholic metabolism, toxic acetaldehyde that builds in her blood also crosses the placenta.

In fact, if the mother drinks too heavily during pregnancy, the baby can suffer fetal alcohol syndrome (FAS). Symptoms include unusual deformities in skull and facial features, mental retardation, severe problems with digestion and metabolism, nervous disorders, malnutrition, and many other extremely serious disorders.

But even if you were born with only a mild addiction to alcohol and begin drinking later in life, alcohol is much more likely to cause you problems. Why? You can reactivate the alcoholic metabolism that developed when you were in the womb.

Advice to pregnant mothers? Don't drink. Current medical advice says don't drink at all during pregnancy. Some studies show that even small amounts of alcohol may compromise fetal health. Also if you are breast-feeding, don't drink, because alcohol passes directly into mother's breast milk.

Sugar addiction. The body metabolizes alcohol and sugar in nearly the same manner. That's why a serious sugar addiction early in life can become the perfect setup for an alcohol addiction later on.

Overconsumption of sweets and other foods high in sugar often leads to hypoglycemia (low blood sugar). Like alcoholism, hypoglycemia is a metabolic problem. And, like alcoholism, it can cause a vicious circle of addiction.

What's the relationship between hypoglycemia and alcoholism? Studies show 95% to 100% of all alcoholic drinkers suffer from hypoglycemia.

Here's what happens: When we ingest sugary foods or alcohol, our blood sugar (glucose) shoots up like a rocket. Blood sugar, you may remember, is a form of food for the cells. It's how the cells get energy. In a strong and healthy body, this energy remains fairly constant. Our cells burn blood sugar at a fairly steady rate, keeping our energy level stable.

We even have built-in controls to ensure this. For instance, when blood sugar rises too quickly, the body undergoes a stress reaction. This immediately signals the pancreas to produce insulin, a hormone that reduces blood sugar. Usually the body produces insulin in just the right amounts, lowering blood sugar to normal levels without much trouble.

After years of excesses and abuse, however, this sugar control system starts to break down. Then the pancreas starts to make mistakes. It begins overreacting. Whenever sugar or alcohol is ingested, it produces too much insulin.

Too much insulin sends the blood sugar level crashing below normal. This abrupt decline results in the body suddenly feeling drained, fatigued, depressed after the initial high. Your energy level goes way down. You may have a headache, feel tense and anxious, or experience fuzzy thinking. These are withdrawal symptoms; they appear anywhere from one to four hours after the initial high. How do you get rid of the symptoms in a hurry? More sweets . . . or alcohol . . . or both.

A hypoglycemic metabolism drives both the sugar and the alcohol addictions. Alcohol relieves you of hypoglycemic symptoms more effectively than sugar. But, as you'd expect, it causes these symptoms to grow more and more severe with each withdrawal.

In fact, alcohol does everything on a slightly grander scale than sugar. It calms you more than sugar because it has a more powerful sedative effect. Yet alcohol also has more toxic side effects than sugar, so the long-range damage to your cells is greater.

Many teenagers exchange their sugar addiction for a more mature addiction: alcohol. The trade-up often happens in adults as well. It's an easy transition because the alcohol addiction fits so neatly into the same biochemical routine as the sugar addiction.

Of course, not all sugar addicts become alcoholic drinkers. But alcohol works wonders for some of them. They instantly prefer it to sweets. For them, alcohol takes the nervous edge off their lives so much more completely. But again, whenever they stop drinking for even a day or two, they keep going for something sweet—often every other hour or so.

When you quit drinking for good, your hypoglycemia can drive you crazy with cravings. Sweets and high-sugar foods will satisfy the cravings temporarily, but not with the supreme calm produced by alcohol.

And if you keep eating sweets or drinking sweet drinks to satisfy the cravings, your metabolism will remain about the same. That means you'll continue to crave alcohol to calm you down.

But if you break your sugar addiction at the same time you quit drinking, you will not crave alcohol. It's actually easier to quit alcohol and sugar together than it is to quit alcohol alone. You'll learn how to do this in Chapter 6.

Overeating. Here's another way you can cause metabolic problems that will set the stage for alcoholism. Overeating, like overdrinking, is a problem of excessive appetite. Many alcoholic drinkers had problems with overeating when they were young, before they started to drink. For some, the habit of overeating disappears when their drinking habit begins. Others alternate habits: they overeat, then they overdrink, then they overeat. Still others do both concurrently.

Interestingly enough, Overeaters Anonymous uses the same 12-step program as AA. However, not enough research has been done to clarify the relationship between these two addictions. More evidence is needed. For now, though, here's an analysis that suggests a biochemical link.

Overeating is a problem of excess, as is alcoholism. Overeating forces the metabolism to work overtime and is especially hard on the liver. The liver has two main functions: to help gain valuable nutrients from normal digestion and to rid the body of toxins. When you eat too much, the liver is forced to work overtime on normal digestion and, as a result, excess toxins accumulate in the blood. The same happens when the liver must process too much alcohol.

Today's food, laced with chemical additives, causes another problem for the overeater. It increases the toxic overload on the liver and can make it even harder for the liver to function properly.

In many ways alcohol brings welcome relief to overeaters. It offers instant calories without the burden of all that digestion. If you drink before you eat, it depresses the appetite and you eat less. If you eat too much and drink afterward, you speed digestion.

Overeating teaches the metabolism how to deal with excess. Overdrinking fits the same biochemical scenario, but it's easier in a way. Why? Alcohol is light; food is heavy. To the overeater, alcohol provides relief while still satisfying the need for excess.

That's why, when you quit drinking, you may naturally begin overeating in order to satisfy your body's expectation for excess. So when you quit, you can do yourself a big favor by learning not to overeat. This in turn will help you to reduce your cravings for alcohol. In Chapter 6, you'll learn how to stop overeating.

Prolonged excessive drinking. Here's one other way normal alcohol metabolism can break down and the alcoholic metabolism begin.

Some habitual drinkers drink a lot without showing serious signs of addiction. But after many years of abuse the internal organs can wear out, especially the pancreas and liver. When the liver loses its ability to metabolize alcohol efficiently, tolerance can increase, and other problems of alcoholism, like excessive cellular damage and withdrawal syndrome, can appear.

This follows the same principle as adult-onset diabetes. The metabolism functions well for a very long time, only to break down after too many years of stress.

Even "social drinkers" and "borderline alcoholics" who average anywhere from two to six drinks per day can experience this phenomenon. All of a sudden things change. They start drinking more and more as addiction sets in.

Prolonged drinking of any amount can trigger hypoglycemia and consequently alcoholism. First, the pancreas breaks down, starting the sugar addiction. Then the liver breaks down, starting the alcohol addiction.

As obvious as this sounds, it doesn't happen very often—at least according to research. Most studies suggest that alcoholic drinkers begin their drinking careers with the metabolic problem already established. Tolerance builds from the very first. Hypoglycemic withdrawal symptoms become slowly exaggerated into more severe alcoholic withdrawal symptoms, along with a greater and greater compulsion to drink.

What Can You Do About the Physical Addiction?

Once started, the physical addiction gets worse and worse. In order to change it, you need to change your metabolism. Here's a quick review:

The alcoholic metabolism drives the physical addiction. This glitch in metabolism boosts the sedative effects of alcohol to your cells. It keeps the body bristling with high doses of sugar to counteract the gloomy side of hypoglycemia. And it creates excess toxins in the body that demand a little extra effort in your own struggle for survival.

Meanwhile, your mind keeps finding all kinds of uses for alcohol. It interprets the way you feel, moment to moment, and knows exactly why you "need another drink." But the mind can't always be trusted. Your body can be near death with alcoholic damage and your mind can want another drink.

But you can change. When you quit drinking and switch to a healthy diet, your cells begin to heal and your metabolism begins to revitalize itself. This is the key. After a while, you begin to feel rejuvenated, strong, and healthy.

A DISEASE CONTROLLED BY DIET

Is alcoholism a disease? There's much confusion.

Pull up a barstool beside any alcoholic drinker and ask whether he thinks he has a disease. He will tell you no, even though he may be quick to admit he's "an alcoholic." But ask any recovering alcoholic in AA. He'll tell you he has a disease and he'll tell you he has this disease whether or not he's drinking.

Each of them is partly right. Alcoholic drinking starts a disease process. This process progresses when you're drinking. It stops when you stop drinking. And when you stop drinking, you can heal much of the damage from the disease if you change your diet.

Alcoholism fits the definition of disease. Like other diseases, alcoholism impairs your health by damaging your cells. Like other diseases, it interrupts your body's vital functions, causing specific symptoms. And like other diseases such as cancer, if it's allowed to continue long enough, it'll kill you.

But as a disease, it has an ironic twist. The agent causing the disease acts like a medicine that cures the symptoms. Alcoholic drinkers actually feel healthier when they're drinking. Pain and sickness seem to disappear. Unfortunately, the sense of health is artificial. When you drink, you relieve yourself of the symptoms only. Meanwhile, inside your body, a disease process rages.

Drinking wears out your body and actually speeds up the aging process. Your cells live their lives in the fast lane of high blood sugar and toxic invaders, grabbing a few thrills but choking on the poisons. You get physically sick more often. Or you feel some slight illness that lingers and is hard to pinpoint.

When cells don't get sufficient nutrients, or if the cells are harmed too often by toxins in the blood, they stop performing important functions. After a while, whole groups of cells begin giving out, and organs begin to fail. Especially susceptible are the brain, heart, liver, pancreas, intestines, kidneys, and stomach.

Metabolism Revisited

The disease itself depends on a problem in metabolism. The problem seems innocent enough. Your liver is simply slow on one step of normal alcohol metabolism: the breakdown of acetaldehyde.

The buildup of acetaldehyde also boosts the brain's production of isoquinoline, a strong sedative similar to morphine or heroin that calms us deeply and kills pain. This added sedative effect greatly increases alcohol's addictive power. It drives us to drink. Thus the damage continues, the disease progresses, and the metabolic problem gets worse.

Metabolism and Diet

Metabolism is intimately connected to diet. Your body metabolizes food for one main purpose: to get vital nutrients to all the cells. To serve this purpose, your body can metabolize many different foods and can learn how to gain nutrients from almost any kind of food you give it. Metabolism also helps rid the body of any unwanted toxins.

Yet your personal metabolism works differently from anyone else's. Studies show that each individual has a unique biochemical makeup and that individuals differ greatly from one another in the way they metabolize various kinds of food. To give you an idea how much possible variation there is, researchers have currently identified over 3,000 metabolic substances (called "metabolites"), and over 1,100 enzymes. Each individual has her own unique proportions of all 4,100 of these biochemicals.

Also, the mixture of biochemicals varies for each kind of food you ingest. For instance, the biochemicals your body produces to metabolize carrots differ somewhat from those it uses for potatoes. Furthermore, your body's biochemicals vary from day to day, and vary depending on what you last ate and even how long ago you ate it.

One more thing: Your body uses quite different biochemicals to metabolize the different classes of foods—meats, grains, vegetables, beans, fruits. As you might have guessed, you need a whole separate biochemical preparedness to handle alcohol, sweets, drugs, chemical additives, and toxins. In fact, too many excesses from this group can cause your metabolism to break down, and begin to make mistakes. For instance, too much sugar too often can cause hypoglycemia. The pancreas begins overreacting (producing too much insulin) when each new burst of sugar hits the bloodstream.

But your body adjusts to whatever diet you give it. The most frequent foods in your diet come to be expected. Biochemical pathways get established the more they are used. Thus, if your body doesn't get an expected food, you actually begin to crave it.

Your body becomes addicted to the foods you give it the most. Your metabolism so completely adjusts to your regular diet that any change from it becomes increasingly difficult. Ask anyone who has attempted a major shift in diet. For instance, if you eat meat regularly, your metabolism will take a long time to adjust to a vegetarian diet. Although the same nutrients are available, your body doesn't have the biochemical preparedness. The ability is there. Your body can metabolize vegetarian meals. But to gain the same efficiency with a new diet can take from one to seven years.

The important thing to remember is this: Metabolism depends on diet. You can change your metabolism if you change your diet. It will take a long time to change your metabolism significantly, but you can feel incredible improvements after just a few months. You'll discover the kind of changes you need to make in Chapter 6.

The Alcoholic Diet

Almost all alcoholic drinkers suffer from malnutrition. Given the amount of alcohol in their diets alone, they don't stand a chance of gaining proper nourishment. Why? Alcohol robs the body of vital nutrients. This happens in two ways:

1. The alcoholic diet leaves little room for nutrient-rich foods. Alcohol is a food itself—with calories but no nutrients. When too many of your calories come from alcohol, you don't have much appetite left for other foods.

2. When you burn calories, your cells require nutrients and burning the "empty calories" of alcohol forces your cells to use reserve nutrients they have stored—especially the B-vitamins and vitamin C. By drinking heavily on just

one occasion, you can completely deplete these reserves.

Alcoholic malnutrition kills slowly. Cells weaken from starvation and become disease-prone. Your behavior can even become bizarre, your thinking impaired. After a while, one of your organs will give out. If it's a vital organ, chances are you'll die.

But if you change your diet, the disease process will stop. The latest research links diet to all major diseases (heart disease, cancer, stroke) and most minor diseases you can think of. But how does diet cause such a long-range debilitating disease as alcoholism? At the root of the dietary problem lies addiction. The alcoholic diet is unbalanced because of various food addictions. The alcohol itself is a dual addiction: a food addiction *and* a drug addiction.

Food addiction, like drug addiction, depends on a biochemical craving. Your body's biochemistry becomes so dependent on a particular food that it grows to expect that food. As with drugs, some foods are more addicting than others. Also, when you stop consuming an addictive food, you experience withdrawal symptoms. These symptoms can be mild, such as headaches, muscle aches, backaches, cramps, diarrhea, constipation, confusion, irregular pulse rate, anxiety, nausea; or more acute, such as dizziness, extreme emotional upset (tears, anger, depression), paranoia, minor convulsions (shakes and tremors), and wild fluctuations in blood pressure.

Nutritionists classify sugar and alcohol as foods because they have calories. This is the only reason for the classification. But as "foods," they are seriously lacking, for neither sugar nor alcohol has any nutrients to help with their digestion. For practical purposes, sugar and alcohol are the same food. One beer has about the same instant caloric value as ten tea-spoons of white sugar.

Among "foods," alcoholic beverages and sugar foods are probably the most addicting you can find. But the additional drug effects of alcohol make it more addicting than sugar. *So when you quit drinking, you must withdraw from both addictions: the food (or sugar) addiction of alcohol and the drug addiction of alcohol.*

You can withdraw from the drug effects in a short time. Depending on the amount of alcohol you drink, severe withdrawal symptoms will last for one to three weeks, and minor symptoms will continue for a few months.

You will begin your withdrawal from the sugar addiction if, when you stop drinking, you stop eating sugar foods as well. In this case, cravings for both sweets and alcohol will diminish after a few weeks, and disappear after six months to a year. If you stop drinking yet continue to eat sugar foods, your hypoglycemia will drive you crazy with regular cravings for alcohol and sweets.

The Cure

Yes, there is a cure for alcoholism.

Your basic goal: to change your metabolism for greater health. That means you need to eliminate alcohol and other addictive foods from your diet and change some other parts of your diet as well.

Then wait.

Why wait? Because once the healing process begins, it takes time to recover. Your body needs time to repair the damage. But the best news is that you begin healing right away. In fact, the healthier your new lifestyle, the faster you will heal. You can heal most of your damaged cells, at least to some degree, because you have your body's replacement policy going for you.

Your body creates new cells every minute—about 300 million to 400 million a day! These new cells replace old and dying cells. When you stop drinking, the new cells your body creates will not be "alcoholic" cells. They will never have tasted alcohol. These new cells will be healthy, if you continue to follow a healthy diet.

Scientists say that every seven years the body replaces every cell (except nerve cells) at least once. That means the body renews itself and becomes a completely new conglomeration of cells. A new you.

This new you begins every day. Now.

CHAPTER 2

Are You an Alcoholic Drinker?

Everything free from falsehood is strength.
—May Sarton

Do you have a problem with alcohol? It's up to you to find out. In this chapter, you will:

- take a closer look at your drinking.
- learn how much you protect your drinking by denying the problems it causes.
- try tests to show whether you're an alcoholic drinker.

I recommend that you start a notebook now. This notebook will be your own private property. You don't have to show it to anyone. Use it to keep track of your life for a while, in order to understand your connection with alcohol. Whenever you have the urge to drink, write down your mood at the time, how you feel about life, how your body feels, what your immediate surroundings are, and what you want to change by drinking. As much as possible, note all the information associated with your drinking habit. Then as you continue to read the self-help methods in this book, you'll discover hundreds of additional ideas to keep you writing.

YOU'RE THE BEST JUDGE

Look at yourself. Basically you know your own condition. Do you feel you have a drinking problem? Somewhere deep inside, you know. Take a look and see what you think.

Here's your first test:

Test #1

One Question

Do you sometimes think you have a drinking problem?

☐ Yes   ☐ No

Your intuition is almost always correct. What you answer is probably true.

But how can a one-question test tell you anything? It's simple. Most of the time, you deny the problem or hide from it by making excuses. It's only natural to protect something so dear to you. But your defenses break down once in a while.

So if you *sometimes* think you have a problem, you almost certainly do.

Imagine yourself the morning after a bad drunk. Your body feels brittle and weak, your defenses shattered. You are completely nauseated and you are in pain. This morning you don't have a morning drink to calm you and, for the moment, you truly feel the misery alcohol is causing you.

This morning you promise yourself you won't drink again. But by the end of the day, your defenses return. You begin to excuse yourself for "one bad night." You didn't eat enough last night, or you were really mad at somebody, or you find some other excuse for having drunk too much. Then you allow yourself to have another drink. You say, "It's okay *now* . . . I was just having a couple of problems *yesterday.*"

You might go through this hundreds of times before you finally recognize the pattern. I know I did.

How can you recognize the pattern of alcoholic drinking? Here's an easy-to-use definition to guide you. Alcoholic drinking is drinking *too much*, *too often*, and *drinking out of control*. Let's look at this three-part definition.

Once again, trust your own judgment. If you feel you're drinking too much and doing it too often, your intuition is probably correct. If you feel it is happening because you can't control it, you are probably addicted. If alcohol eliminates your self-control, or if your drinking alters your personality, you almost certainly have a problem.

Pay attention to your deepest feelings. Try writing them in your notebook. Write how you feel about your drinking, how you feel about how much and how often you drink, and what kind of control you have over it. You don't need to analyze it. Just say what you feel . . . it may surprise you.

STOP HIDING

> *He who conceals his disease cannot expect to be cured.*
> —*Ethiopian proverb*

Alcoholic drinkers like drinking so much, they'll do almost anything to protect it. Do you protect your drinking habit? When problems arise from your drinking, do you try to deny them or minimize them? There are three main ways you may be protecting your drinking:

1. You may deny how serious the problems are.
2. You may deny that alcohol causes the problems.
3. You may make excuses for your drinking.

Alcoholic drinkers use all three methods to hide from reality. You'll find a list of specific denials and excuses people use in Worksheet #1, at the end of this section.

Each alcoholic drinker has an elaborate system of denials and excuses. Georgia denied her problems with alcohol and made excuses to suit her needs. In fact, she enjoyed the challenge of it. Whenever anyone suggested she had a problem with her drinking, she had another excuse. It was like playing a chess game—and she was very good at staying one move ahead of her opponent. But this kept her from the truth for a very long time. Almost too long. When she finally got a medical checkup, she found that her physical condition was extremely serious, much worse than she ever admitted to anyone (including herself).

Your denials and excuses to others are alarming enough, but they become even worse when you start believing them yourself. When that happens, it means you can maintain a false image of your health for a long time. Meanwhile, problems inside you can be raging out of control, and getting worse. Problems all around you—with family, romantic relationships, friendships—can become more extreme as well. That's why it's important to break this pattern as soon as you can.

How do you break the pattern? One way is to wait

until you get a big scare, a near-death experience caused by alcoholic drinking—something so obvious you simply cannot deny it. It can be a severe health crisis, an accident, or something you did while drunk that you very much regret. A big scare dissolves all lies. Almost instantly you can see directly into your own reality.

But if you do have a problem with alcohol, this is not the best way to find out. Don't wait to get a jolt like this, because you may not survive it.

The other way to break the pattern—the best way—is to simply stop the lies. Then you can see the real you and the real problems alcohol causes in you. Once you can detect the lies, you can stop them. The following worksheet will help you.

Worksheet #1

Denials and Excuses

Instructions: Look over the following lists and check the denials and excuses you use. Return to it periodically for a few weeks to a couple of months, to make sure you don't miss anything. Add your own excuses if you don't find them listed here, in the exact wording. When you know the exact words you use, you can see more clearly what you're trying to hide. Go over your list now and then, until you feel it's complete. (Work here, on this page, or work in your notebook.)

Denials

Denying Seriousness of Problems

☐ I'm not addicted . . . I can stop whenever I want.

☐ I don't have any problems with alcohol. My drinking isn't a problem.

☐ I'm using alcohol for a good purpose. It helps me with

_____ .

☐ Alcohol is like a medicine to me.

☐ I don't drink too much. Just a few drinks now and then. (Check here if you use this lie to convince others that you don't drink too much. Check here also if you hide liquor or sneak drinks.)

☐ Sure I might drink a lot . . . but alcohol never gets the best of me.

☐ I can always make it to work on time (or: I can always get the meals cooked and the clothes washed, or anything that suggests you fulfill your responsibilities in spite of your drinking).

☐ (Referring to any kind of internal problem): It's just a little pain . . . It usually goes away when I take a drink.

☐ Well, I made it home all right, so everything must be okay (or: I didn't get picked up by the police, so I must've driven okay. Then you look at your car and see a scrape: Well, it's only a scrape . . . there's no blood, so it's okay).

☐ It was an accident. Accidents happen to everybody.

☐ It's just a minor problem . . . it doesn't do too much harm.

☐ Other ways you deny the seriousness of alcohol-related problems:

_____

_____

_____

_____

_____

_____

_____

_____

_____

Denying Alcohol Causes the Problems

☐ I was nervous as hell . . . I simply had to have a drink. (Instead of realizing the nervous tension was caused by alcohol withdrawal.)

☐ I was feeling so down . . . I needed a pick-me-up. (Also denying your feelings were caused by alcohol withdrawal.)

☐ I was really upset . . . so I went to the bar to have a few. (Once again, denying a sign of withdrawal.)

☐ It's not alcohol that makes me this way. It's just me. It's the way I am.

☐ It's not the alcohol that's messing me up. My life's a little crazy, that's all.

☐ It's not the alcohol . . . I've never gotten ahead in life because I don't come from a privileged background.

☐ I didn't lose the job because of drinking. That job wasn't "my style" . . . and I never liked it anyway.

☐ These troubles have just started happening lately. I don't know where they come from.

☐ It's not my drinking . . . it's something else. (I just haven't been eating well lately. Or: I'm under a lot of pressure lately. Or: _____ .)

☐ Stay out of my business. It's my life and you don't know anything about what's wrong with me (whenever someone suggests you have a drinking problem).

☐ It's not the alcohol. It's the cigarettes (or: the coffee, or: that damned drug I'm taking).

☐ I must be constipated (or: have diarrhea) because of the food I ate (not because of my drinking).

☐ Gee, this pain in my right side (liver) is really bothering me. I wonder what's wrong.

   You can use this denial with many physical symptoms, pretending alcohol has nothing to do with them.

   ☐ This pain in the middle of my back (kidneys).

   ☐ This pain in my left side (pancreas).

   ☐ My high blood pressure.

   ☐ That damned ulcer.

☐   My unclear thinking.

☐   _____ (See Worksheet #3 in Chapter 3 for other problems alcohol causes that you might be denying.)

☐ Other ways you deny that alcohol causes problems:

_____

_____

_____

_____

_____

_____

_____

Excuses

Excuses to Start Drinking

☐ I need a drink to unwind.

☐ I'm having a rough day . . . I think I'll have a drink.

☐ Whenever _____ (wife/husband/girlfriend/boyfriend/boss/friend/son/daughter/mother/father) gets mad at me, I just want to get drunk.

☐ It's happy hour (cocktail hour, attitude adjustment hour) . . . time to have a drink.

☐ I had a bad day.

☐ I had a good day.

☐ The sun is shining.

☐ It's cloudy and miserable.

☐ It's cold out! I need a drink to warm me up.

☐ It's hot out! I need a drink to cool me down.

☐ I worked hard . . . got a lot done. Now I'll reward myself.

☐ I'm thirsty . . . I need a drink.

☐ I need some hair of the dog that bit me.

☐ I need an eye-opener.

☐ I need a drink to give me a lift.

☐ It helps me put up with some unbearable situation:

☐ I need a drink to _____ .
(Fill in the blank with your reasons for drinking. See
Worksheet #2 for help. Your reasons for drinking can
quickly become excuses for drinking.)

☐ Other excuses you use to start drinking:

_____

_____

_____

_____

_____

_____

_____

Excuses to Continue Drinking

☐ I need one more to settle me down.

☐ Well . . . I'm started now.

☐ You only live once . . . so you might as well go for it!

☐ Well, if you're buying.

☐ I need another drink to keep going.

☐ What the hell. Sure, I'll have another one.

☐ I need one more to really have a good time.

☐ I need one more to face _____ (a certain
person), or be with _____ (a certain person).

☐ I need one more to get in the mood . . . to get just the
right buzz . . . just the right glow.

☐ One more to get rid of this anger (or: any other bad
emotion).

☐ One for the road.

☐ One to good friends.

☐ Here's to your health.

☐ All right, if you insist.

☐ Just one more.

☐ A nightcap.

☐ Other excuses you use to keep drinking, once you start:

_____

_____

_____

_____

_____

_____

_____

Excuses for Drinking Too Much

☐ I guess I had one (or two, or a few) too many last night.

☐ It's not my fault. They kept buying me drinks. What was I to do?

☐ I shouldn't have drunk on an empty stomach.

☐ I got drunk because I mixed my drinks (or: because I drank hard stuff instead of beer).

☐ I couldn't help it. It was just one of those things. I simply drank too much and that's that.

☐ My drinking isn't the problem . . . I drank too much because of my real problem: _____ .

☐ I was under too much stress and alcohol helped me forget.

☐ Sorry, I won't get that way again.

☐ I just forgot to watch how much I drank.

☐ Damn it all! I'll never get that drunk again.

☐ After last night, I never want to touch the stuff. I'm going to quit it for good.

☐ What the hell . . . I just drank too much. It's not the end of the world.

☐ So-and-so, _____ , was worse off than I was.

☐ This time I finally learned my lesson.

☐ Don't worry, it'll pass.

☐ It wasn't my fault . . . I was just too drunk to know what I was doing. (Excuses like this get more serious. Instead of excusing overdrinking, you excuse bad behavior because of overdrinking; for instance, after beating your spouse or child, you say, "It wasn't my fault . . . I just drank too much.")

☐ Hey, we really tied a good one on last night, didn't we?

☐ Wow! I really got wasted last night . . . but what a night.

☐ It'll make a good story, won't it?

☐ I don't remember anything. It's a complete blank.

☐ I'm sorry if I said anything to offend you.

☐ I'm sorry I hit you. The alcohol made me do it.

☐ I hope I didn't make any enemies last night, or hurt anybody. No . . . I couldn't have . . . could I?

☐ If I just apologize for being drunk, everything will be okay.

☐ Other excuses you use for drinking too much:

_____

_____

_____

_____

_____

_____

_____

_____

_____

NOW TAKE ANOTHER LOOK

> *Nothing can be loved or hated unless it is first known.*
>
> —*Leonardo da Vinci*

A number of recent Mayo Clinic studies have shown that "paper and pencil" tests identify alcoholic drinkers more consistently and more accurately than laboratory tests. It seems the lab tests aren't sensitive enough to catch all the cases. Those who had passed their physical tests but showed signs of alcoholism on their written tests were checked again. Almost invariably the written test proved correct.

Test #2 can show whether you have a problem with alcohol. You'll also learn a little about how bad the problem really is. This test has become a standard in the field.

Give it a try.

Test #2

The Johns Hopkins Medical Institution's Test for Alcoholism

This test was originated at Johns Hopkins University, Department of Psychiatry and Behavioral Sciences, The Blades Center, 550 N. Broadway, Suite 202, Baltimore, MD 21205 (phone 410-955-6901).

Instructions: Answer the questions honestly. Then score yourself according to the key. Work here or in your notebook.

	YES	NO
1. Do you lose time from work due to drinking?	☐	☐

	YES	NO
2. Is drinking making your home life unhappy?	☐	☐
3. Do you drink because you are shy with other people?	☐	☐
4. Is drinking affecting your reputation?	☐	☐
5. Have you ever felt remorse after drinking?	☐	☐
6. Have you gotten into financial difficulties as a result of drinking?	☐	☐
7. Do you turn to lower companions and an inferior environment when drinking?	☐	☐
8. Does your drinking make you careless of your family's welfare?	☐	☐
9. Has your ambition decreased since drinking?	☐	☐
10. Do you crave a drink at a definite time daily?	☐	☐
11. Do you want a drink the next morning?	☐	☐
12. Does drinking cause you difficulty in sleeping?	☐	☐
13. Has your efficiency decreased since drinking?	☐	☐
14. Is drinking jeopardizing your job or business?	☐	☐
15. Do you drink to escape from worries or trouble?	☐	☐
16. Do you drink alone?	☐	☐
17. Have you ever had a complete loss of memory because of drinking?	☐	☐
18. Has your physician ever treated you for drinking?	☐	☐
19. Do you drink to build up your self-confidence?	☐	☐
20. Have you ever been to a hospital or institution on account of drinking?	☐	☐

> If you have answered yes to any one of the questions, there is a definite warning that you may be an alcoholic. If you have answered yes to any two, the chances are that you are an alcoholic. If you have answered yes to three or more, you are definitely an alcoholic.

You may want to try another test from the National Council on Alcoholism and Drug Dependence, the NCADD Self-Test, which is also considered a valuable test in the field. To request a copy, write to NCADD, 12 W. 21st Street, New York, NY·10010; or call 800-NCA-CALL.

WHAT'S THE VERDICT?

To understand is to forgive, even oneself.
—*Alexander Chase*

Now that you've taken a closer look, you should know more about your relationship with alcohol. What did you learn? After carefully considering your relationship to alcohol, have you decided to do anything about it? What have you decided to do?

As your next step, in Chapter 3 you'll discover more about alcohol-related problems—and which ones affect you the most. You'll also judge for yourself how serious your problems have become.

If you have a problem with alcohol, remember this: you can handle it. You'll learn plenty of ways to help yourself. But if you feel you need to quit drinking right away, do Checklist #1 in Chapter 3 and read the section just after that to determine whether you need in-patient care for detox. Then quit. You can just as easily do the remaining techniques in Chapters 3 through 8 after you quit drinking.

CHAPTER 3

Are the Benefits Worth the Problems?

He who hesitates is sometimes saved.
—James Thurber

Take a moment to consider: How bad is your problem with alcohol? How many things have gone wrong in your life since you first started heavy drinking?

You may have some trouble answering these two questions. Why? Because you keep remembering the benefits you get from drinking. Alcohol helps you cope in so many ways, you tend to overlook the problems it causes. You may deny the problems. Or you may not realize that alcohol is causing many of your problems.

Actually, alcohol has many side effects. When you drink too much, every living cell in your body is harmed. In a short time the damage becomes very serious. Your vital organs weaken: your heart, your brain, your liver, your digestive organs, your sex organs. Because of this, you tend to have thought disorders, heart disease, skin problems, digestive problems, weak bones, sexual dysfunction (including problems with childbirth), nervous disorders, and emotional problems. Furthermore, as your cells become weaker, you become more susceptible to degenerative diseases like cancer and AIDS.

In this chapter you'll weigh the benefits of alcohol against the problems it causes and decide whether you need to quit drinking. Even if you have already decided to quit, these exercises will help you to confirm and to strengthen your reasons for quitting.

Back in the early days of AA—until the mid-1960s—it was said that alcoholics had to hit "rock bottom" before they could begin to change. With early self-assessment (from the checklists and worksheets in this chapter), however, you can decide to make a change before you hit rock bottom, and in turn save yourself a lot of trouble. Things might be bad now, but you can decide to change before they get worse.

As your first step, take a look at the many different ways you use alcohol to help you cope.

THE BENEFITS OF DRINKING

> What does drunkenness not accomplish? It
> unlocks secrets, confirms our hopes, urges the
> indolent into battle, lifts the burden from
> anxious minds, teaches new arts.
> —Horace

Alcohol may be hurting you, but you keep drinking because it also does something good for you. You use alcohol to gain certain benefits in life. Ask anybody who drinks heavily and he or she can give you plenty of good reasons for drinking.

What are your reasons? Do Worksheet #2 to find out.

Worksheet #2

My Reasons for Drinking

Instructions: Put a check next to each one of your reasons for drinking. Check as many reasons as you feel relate to you. Use the blank lines in each category to write any additional reasons you have.

To forget about myself or my problems:

☐ It helps me stop worrying.

☐ It helps reduce tension.

☐ It helps me relax or wind down.

☐ It helps when I'm depressed.

☐ It helps when I feel lonely.

☐ It helps me forget my problems.

☐ It helps me feel better when everything seems hopeless.

☐ Alcohol helps when I feel nobody cares about me.

☐ It helps me avoid painful memories (drown my sorrows).

☐ Sometimes I drink when I feel guilty or ashamed (even when it's my drinking I feel guilty or ashamed about).

☐ It helps me forget a serious crisis in my life, such as losing a loved one, a bad accident, getting fired (write it here): _____

☐ _____

☐ _____

For pleasure, kicks, or the thrill of it:

☐ When I drink, I feel I have more fun.

☐ Sometimes I drink to celebrate. (It can be anything: a holiday, good news, a reunion with an old friend.)

☐ Sometimes I drink for sentimental reasons . . . to remember something pleasurable in the past.

☐ I drink because I like the taste of certain drinks.

☐ I like the effects of getting high. I like the glow.

☐ I like the taste of alcoholic beverages with certain foods I eat.

☐ Just for kicks.

☐ _____

☐ _____

To reduce inhibitions, make me feel more powerful, or help me get along with others:

☐ When I drink, I don't feel so shy.

☐ It helps me in social situations.

☐ I feel I perform better sexually.

☐ It helps me express my anger.

☐ Sometimes I drink just to show people I can drink (especially if they've been telling me they think I should quit).

☐ It shows how tough I am. You gotta be tough to drink as much as I can.

☐ It makes me feel more mature.

☐ It helps me speak my mind.

☐ It helps me face responsibilities.

☐ It builds my courage.

☐ It helps me take risks.

☐ It helps me accept failure when things don't work out.

☐ When I drink I feel more complete, more fulfilled.

☐ It makes me feel more loving.

☐ When I drink, I feel more independent.

☐ _____

☐ _____

To sedate me:

- ☐ When I drink, I don't feel so nervous.
- ☐ It helps me sleep.
- ☐ It helps stop the shakes in the morning.
- ☐ Drinking gets rid of pain (headache, muscle pain, toothache, cramps, any other body ache or pain).
- ☐ It stops me from thinking too much.
- ☐ It helps when I'm feeling stressed.
- ☐ It slows me down when things seem to be going too fast.
- ☐ _____
- ☐ _____

To stimulate me:

- ☐ It picks me up when I'm feeling down.
- ☐ It rouses me when I feel bored.
- ☐ It helps me wake up in the morning (an eye-opener).
- ☐ It helps clear my head.
- ☐ It helps me be more creative.
- ☐ _____
- ☐ _____

It's automatic, part of my lifestyle:

- ☐ I drink because other people expect me to drink (especially at certain times: at recreational activities, at lunch, on the job, at happy hour).
- ☐ It's the only way I know. It's my lifestyle.
- ☐ It's automatic. Sometimes I start drinking without even realizing it.
- ☐ It's part of my life. I'm attached to it . . . I'd be completely lost without it.
- ☐ _____
- ☐ _____

To satisfy my addiction; to avoid unpleasant feelings of withdrawal:

☐ I can go only a certain amount of time before I need a drink.

☐ Sometimes I drink to stop myself from being hungry.

☐ Often I feel as if I just have to have a drink.

☐ When I stop drinking, I start feeling sick.

☐ I drink because I don't have a choice . . . I'm seriously addicted to alcohol.

☐ It helps kill an irresistible urge for alcohol—a deep craving inside my gut.

☐ My drinking stops this cold, clammy feeling I sometimes get when I haven't had a drink for a while.

☐ It stops the DTs (severe trembling, hallucinations, seizures).

☐ _____

☐ _____

Now take a second look. Maybe you remember using alcohol to calm you down. When you drink, alcohol does sedate you. But as the alcohol leaves your system, you become more agitated than before you started drinking. Over time it takes more and more alcohol to calm you because withdrawal from alcohol makes you more and more agitated. You have to stay drunk all the time or drink until you're nearly passed out before you finally feel calm.

Maybe you said you use alcohol to help you have fun. Now when you drink you don't really have fun. You have memories of fun. Maybe your drinking has become so serious that it's simply not really fun anymore.

Maybe you said drinking helps you have better sex. But now your drinking often kills your desire, impairs your ability, or makes you pass out before you can even have sex.

After a while alcohol stops helping you with specific problems, or else you need more and more to overcome these problems. Instead of one drink now, it may take two or three drinks to stop the shakes, or to keep you from feeling sick, or to hold off the DTs.

In fact, you may find that alcohol doesn't help you at all anymore. But you continue drinking because you remember how it helped you in the past. Many folks keep drinking for years in an attempt to recreate "the good days." But those days never return.

Now go back over your list and put *a second check* next to anything that alcohol *still* helps you do. Think about each benefit and be honest with yourself. Ask, "Does alcohol still help me do this?"

Undoubtedly you feel alcohol does still help you in certain ways: some of the items on your list probably have two checks. But, in order to quit drinking successfully, you need to find other ways to do what alcohol does for you now. The remaining chapters offer you successful methods to gain the benefits of drinking without the drinking.

PROBLEMS CAUSED BY DRINKING

How can you get a clear picture of alcohol's true value in your life? You just looked at the benefits. Now compare them with some of the problems alcohol causes.

A few years ago a friend of mine died of cirrhosis. She had been a heavy, daily drinker for 16 years. I liked Sarah very much. She was a happy-go-lucky person who laughed and joked a lot. She left behind a husband and two teenage daughters when she died at age 38.

What a tragedy! Why hadn't she taken the time to evaluate her condition? If Sarah had gotten a medical checkup a couple of years earlier, it could have saved her life. Knowing alcohol would kill her, she could have finally decided to quit drinking and begun to heal herself.

How can anyone let a problem go this far? Is it because most of us tend to overlook our problems?

Originally you started drinking in order to gain something. You got certain benefits. But soon you started drinking in order to escape problems or forget about how bad you feel. Unfortunately, too much alcohol makes your problems even worse and it becomes a vicious circle, a self-defeating mechanism. The very way you choose to solve your problems actually aggravates and intensifies them.

What's worse, your drinking causes its own problems—problems that become so serious they can kill you. Be assured that alcoholic drinking will kill you, sooner or later. It's slow suicide for some and fast suicide for others.

One recovering drinker, Billie Jean, told me, "It's like being married to someone you love very much, then finding out that person is a beast who's trying to kill you." At some point you'll discover that alcohol is a beast that's trying to kill you. And at that moment your love affair will end.

But, for the time being, you keep the benefits of drinking in your mind. You *know* them. You *think* about them often. You can put them into words. The problems drinking causes remain in the body, just under the surface. They're not so obvious and, chances are, you haven't put them into words. You don't usually think about them or talk about them. Even so, you can find these problems if you take a look. In this section, you'll take a look.

Is Alcohol Hurting You More Than You Know?

Most people realize that too much alcohol harms their bodies. But how much harm does it do? Practice #1 helps you break through your denials and look at alcohol's potential threat to your physical health.

Your body holds many secrets. As alcohol compromises your health, your body sends warning signs. Unfortunately, too many drinkers make the mistake of ignoring these important signs.

So here's your chance to unlock these inner secrets. Just take some time and listen to your body.

You'll find this exercise works best when you're not drinking. It can be particularly effective when you have a serious hangover.

Practice #1

Dialogue with Body

Close your eyes. Relax. Get as comfortable as you possibly can.

Now go inside yourself and practice centering your attention on different parts of your body. By projecting your mind into your body, you can determine how it feels. Ask your body to tell you how it responds to alcohol. Let your mind center in different organs, glands, and muscles and, as you do, be sensitive to their condition. Ask each part, "How do you feel about alcohol? How does alcohol affect you?" Ask:

your feet
your legs
your back
your chest
your hands
your arms
your face
your head

You may touch these areas with your hand as you center your mind on them.

Then allow different organs, and organ groups, to tell you how they feel about alcohol:

> your heart
> your liver (right side at bottom of rib cage)
> your pancreas (left side at bottom of rib cage)
> your throat
> your stomach
> your intestines
> your kidneys (middle of back, both sides)
> your sex organs (organs of reproduction)
> your lungs
> your brain

Again, it helps to touch these areas with your hands as you think about them.

Finally, ask your five senses how they feel about alcohol:

> your eyesight (you may open your eyes a few times for this one)
> your hearing
> your sense of touch
> your sense of smell
> your sense of taste

Take as much time as possible with each area of your body. Listen as long as you can before moving on. This may not be easy at first, but be patient. Your body will soon open up to you.

Write your responses in your notebook, or use a separate sheet of paper. I suggest putting your comments in writing because it will help you remember them.

I started doing Practice #1 about a year before I quit drinking. What a discovery! I learned how much my body really hated alcohol. I'd been aching and hurting from drinking for years. My body wanted to quit drinking. Later, when I finally did quit, it helped me very much to know that some major part of me desperately wanted to make a change.

My body knew the problems alcohol was causing. It was my mind that loved alcohol. It was my mind that forced me to drink. My mind had simply been ignoring my body all those years.

The part of you that's alcoholic lives in the mind. Your body can be ailing and weeping, yet your mind can still want a drink. When you quit drinking, it helps to get in touch with your body—to get your mind listening to your body more often.

Alcohol and Your Health

In this section, you'll discover the specific medical problems alcohol causes. You can discern many of these problems by yourself, but you should plan on getting a physical checkup, which will let you know for sure whether you have a medical condition and how serious it is.

As your first step, you need to find the right physician. You want one who knows addictions, especially alcohol addiction. So ask around. Often the best place to go is an alcoholism clinic. You don't have to admit yourself for treatment; tell them you just want a medical assessment.

Then plan to tell the doctor everything. First off, state that you're concerned about your drinking. Describe as much about your drinking history as the doctor wants to know. Be as accurate as possible. In addition, report how you scored on the tests in Chapter 2.

Checklist #1 gives you a fairly complete list of signs, disorders, and diseases common to alcoholic drinkers. As an alcoholic drinker, you run a greater risk than normal of getting every one of them. If you have any of them already, it may indicate serious trouble. Even simple visible signs often indicate a deeper problem. For instance, red skin blemishes are associated with liver malfunction.

Checklist #1

Checklist of Medical Problems

Instructions: Three steps. (1) Look over the following list of symptoms. Put a check next to any symptom you have now, or have had in the past five years. (2) Share the list with a doctor. These symptoms are signs of deeper problems, so be sure to get tested to determine what deeper problems you might have. (3) What problems do you have? Look over the list of medical problems common to alcoholic drinkers. Check the problems that have been diagnosed in you.

Symptoms

Liver/Gallbladder

☐ sensitivity in right abdomen (push two or three fingers into right abdomen, just below ribs)

☐ pains in right abdomen

☐ hardened, enlarged area in right abdomen

☐ yellowing of skin, yellow whites of eyes, or a tan on a light-skinned person even without sun (jaundice)

☐ vomiting blood

Pancreas/Spleen

☐ sensitivity in left abdomen just below ribs

☐ pains in left abdomen

Gastrointestinal

☐ frequent sore throat

☐ swelling of abdomen with fluid, "beer belly" (ascites)

☐ stomach pain

☐ stomach cramps

- ☐ abdominal pain with meals
- ☐ frequent heartburn
- ☐ digestive problems
- ☐ frequent vomiting
- ☐ bowel problems: diarrhea, constipation, or diarrhea alternating with constipation
- ☐ bloody or black stools

Kidneys and Bladder

- ☐ pains on either side of the middle of back
- ☐ cramps in the middle of the back
- ☐ difficulty or pain urinating

Metabolism

- ☐ excessive hunger
- ☐ excessive thirst
- ☐ frequent headaches
- ☐ craving sweets
- ☐ excessive urination (more than four or five times a day)
- ☐ shakiness or nervous tension, especially just before eating
- ☐ feeling weak
- ☐ cold, clammy feeling
- ☐ feeling jittery
- ☐ confused thinking

Lungs

- ☐ excessive congestion
- ☐ frequent colds

Heart

- ☐ chest pains
- ☐ swelling in feet
- ☐ rapid heartbeat (tachycardia)

- [ ] rapid, irregular heartbeat (palpitations)
- [ ] abnormal changes in heartbeat (arrythmia)

Blood

- [ ] extreme weakness
- [ ] feeling faint
- [ ] occasional fainting

Joints, Muscles, and Bones

- [ ] sore joints
- [ ] sharp pain in joints
- [ ] frequent broken bones
- [ ] muscle cramps
- [ ] muscle pains
- [ ] poor muscle development or tone

Eyes

- [ ] dimness of vision, particularly night vision
- [ ] poor vision or problems with vision
- [ ] repeated eye infections

Sex Organs

- [ ] decrease in size of testicles
- [ ] increased vaginal infections
- [ ] decreased sex drive (male or female)
- [ ] decreased enjoyment of sex

Skin

- [ ] general redness or flushing
- [ ] small red blemishes in spiderlike pattern (blemishes turn white with pressure)
- [ ] increase of visible red blood vessels on face
- [ ] prominent veins on belly
- [ ] an enlarged red nose

- ☐ red acne-type skin (rosacea)
- ☐ dark red blotches
- ☐ permanent reddish-blue mottling especially on the hands or feet (livedo reticularis)
- ☐ poor skin condition in general
- ☐ ulcers of the skin

Other General Signs

- ☐ poor hair condition
- ☐ loss of hair
- ☐ hoarseness
- ☐ increased gag reflex (back of tongue at esophagus)
- ☐ bleeding gums
- ☐ sores on the body
- ☐ clubbing of fingers
- ☐ bags or circles under eyes
- ☐ steady weight loss or steady weight gain
- ☐ overdevelopment of mammary glands in males
- ☐ frequent accidents

Nervous and Mental Disorders

- ☐ feeling on edge, jumpy
- ☐ nervous tension
- ☐ shooting pains in extremities
- ☐ extreme weakness
- ☐ forgetfulness
- ☐ memory loss
- ☐ loss of normal logical thinking ability
- ☐ loss of coordination
- ☐ clouded thinking
- ☐ exaggerated reaction to a stimulus (either too slow or too quick)
- ☐ hallucinations (seeing, hearing, feeling, smelling, or tasting things that are not there)

☐ tremors, mild to severe
☐ convulsions, seizures, delirium tremens (DTs)

Emotional Warning Signals

☐ moodiness
☐ frequent crying
☐ family problems
☐ interpersonal problems
☐ work-related problems
☐ suicidal thoughts

Medical Problems (Diagnosed)

Liver/Gallbladder

☐ fatty liver (precursor to cirrhosis)
☐ hepatitis (inflammation of the liver)
☐ cancer of the liver or gallbladder
☐ cirrhosis (long onset but once started proceeds rapidly; biggest killer of alcoholic drinkers: about 14,000 a year)

Pancreas/Spleen

☐ pancreatitis (inflammation of the pancreas)
☐ cancer of the pancreas or spleen

Gastrointestinal

☐ ulcers, recurring or nonhealing
☐ esophagitis (inflammation of esophagus)
☐ cancer of esophagus
☐ gastritis (inflammation of the stomach)
☐ inflammations of the intestines (colitis, Crohn's disease, and others)
☐ cancer of the intestines, especially of the colon and rectum

Kidneys and Bladder

☐ chronic bladder infections
☐ cancer of the bladder
☐ kidney failure

Metabolism

☐ hypoglycemia (low blood sugar, common to all alcoholic drinkers)
☐ diabetes (hyperglycemia: excessive amounts of sugar in the blood)

Lungs

☐ bronchitis
☐ frequent pneumonia
☐ lung cancer

Heart

☐ hypertension (high blood pressure)
☐ myocardiopathy (disease of the heart muscle)
☐ congestive heart failure

Blood

☐ anemia (deficiency of red blood cells causing extreme weakness, sometimes fainting)

Joints, Muscles, and Bones

☐ osteoporosis (bones lose mass and become brittle)
☐ gout (inflammation of joints caused by imbalance of uric acid metabolism)
☐ myopathies (various diseases of the muscle)

Eyes

☐ various inflammations of the eye
☐ lateral nystagmus (jerking movement of eyes with gaze to the left or right)

Sex Organs

☐ male impotence
☐ frequent urinary tract infections
☐ various inflammations of uterus

Skin

☐ skin cancer

Vitamin Deficiency Diseases

☐ malnutrition
☐ neuritis (inflammation of the nerves; most common: peripheral neuritis affecting nerves in the limbs)
☐ toxic amblyopia (dimness of vision caused by toxic effects of alcohol)
☐ beriberi (nervous disorder due primarily to lack of vitamin B1)
☐ pellagra (caused by vitamin B3 deficiency, resulting in skin eruptions, problems with digestion, nervous system disturbances, and eventual psychosis)
☐ scurvy (caused by vitamin C deficiency, leading to bleeding gums, serious internal bleeding, and extreme weakness)

Nervous and Mental Disorders

☐ neuropathies (any of various disorders or diseases of the nervous system)
☐ convulsive disorders
☐ degenerative nerve diseases
☐ Wernicke's syndrome (mental disorder involving loss of coordination and disruption of the senses; symptoms include memory loss, disorientation, agitation, and confusion)

☐ Korsakoff's syndrome or alcohol amnesic disorder (thought disorder due to brain deterioration; symptoms include disruption of memory, memory loss, inability to process information, extreme agitation, hallucinations, and loss of normal logical thinking; about 66% of those with Korsakoff's syndrome can never recover, and up to 17% die in the acute phase of this disorder)

You may have one or more of these problems. The more of these problems you have, the more you stand to gain when you quit drinking.

When you quit drinking, your body begins to heal itself. If these conditions haven't gotten too serious, you can improve them, if not reverse them completely.

WILL YOU NEED INPATIENT CARE?

Alcohol withdrawal is serious business. Of those who go it alone, without medical treatment, 20% to 25% die in acute convulsions. The critical phase can last from 3 to 14 days. You must determine ahead of time how severe your alcohol withdrawal will be and whether you will need inpatient care when you quit.

What does inpatient care mean? It means going to a hospital or detoxification center (some detox centers are located in hospitals). The detox team will help you get over the hardest part of quitting: withdrawal. You go in drunk and come out sober. The length of stay can be anywhere from 5 to 30 days. Most units offer 24-hour supervision during severe withdrawal. A variety of additional services may be offered to help with your recovery.

A doctor familiar with alcoholism can tell you whether you will need inpatient care. Ask the doctor you've chosen to give you your checkup. But if you don't go to a doctor to find out and *if you're in doubt, the answer is: Yes, you will need inpatient care when you quit.*

You know your alcoholism better than anybody else. Do you begin to have serious problems whenever you go without alcohol for more than a day? If so, plan to use an inpatient center for detox.

Look around. There are hundreds of centers available. You can probably find four or five near you. Check each one and ask questions about how they operate. Then pick the one you feel is right for you.

When you go, plan to participate with the staff and other patients. You will learn a lot by doing so. And when you go, take this book with you. That way you can continue to develop your own successful program for quitting. The rest of this book contains hundreds of suggestions that will help you do this.

YOUR EVALUATION OF THE PROBLEMS

In the last chapter, you learned how you deny many of your problems related to alcohol. In this chapter, so far, you have searched inside yourself to identify some of these problems. You also had a thorough medical checkup.

Now it's time to use the information you have gained . . . and make sure you don't deny anything.

Worksheet #3

Problems You'd Like to Avoid

Instructions: Here you'll find a list of problems not mentioned in previous sections. Check any that bother you. At the end of the list, in the blank lines, write any health problems you discovered from your medical checkup. Also make sure to include anything you learned from your own inner search.

I want to avoid:

☐ loss of self-control.

☐ taking too many risks. I could seriously injure or even kill myself or someone else in an accident.

☐ dying younger. (Alcoholic drinkers die 12 to 15 years younger than nondrinkers.)

☐ violence. Alcohol makes me violent. I could hurt someone I love. Or I could hurt someone I don't even know.

☐ being overweight. Alcohol makes me fat.

☐ fetal alcohol syndrome. (Alcoholic drinking while pregnant causes serious disabilities in your child. The best way to look at it: If you want to drink, don't have a baby; if you want to have a baby, don't drink.)

☐ looking older than I am. (Excessive drinking accelerates aging. The effects can be seen on the skin.)

☐ problems with sex.

☐ losing my sexiness. (In the male, alcoholic drinking causes impotence, inability to get an erection. In the female, orgasms become weaker or disappear.)

☐ feeling like I'm a failure.

☐ tension.

☐ anxiety.

☐ mental confusion. I can't think clearly, or I can't make up my mind about things.

☐ feeling bad about myself.

☐ feeling too dependent on alcohol.

☐ feeling too dependent on other people.

☐ hurting my ability to love. (Alcohol destroys loving relationships.)

☐ feeling lost. I feel I don't have any sense of spiritual connection with the world.

☐ feeling lonely.

☐ losing good friends because of alcohol.

☐ planning too much of my life around alcohol.

☐ feeling like I'm losing my mind. (Actual memory loss does occur with excessive drinking.)

☐ feeling too much pain and physical discomfort.

☐ fighting for control of my life.

☐ dulling my sense of taste.

☐ dulling my sense of smell.

☐ depression.

☐ nervousness.

☐ feeling like I might commit suicide. (Alcoholic drinkers are 6 to 15 times more likely to commit suicide than moderate drinkers and nondrinkers.)

☐ greater likelihood of accident while driving. (Drunken driving is the leading cause of death among young people ages 16 to 24. Drivers with blood alcohol levels above 0.10 percent are 3 to 15 times more likely to have a fatal accident than nondrinkers.)

☐ irregular menstrual cycle.

☐ infertility (women).

☐ higher rate of miscarriages.

☐ legal problems: various alcohol-related arrests.

☐ financial worries: too much money spent on alcohol and alcohol-related problems.

☐ difficulty keeping a job.

☐ losing self-esteem.

☐ feeling like people don't care about me anymore.

☐ feeling like everything is hopeless.

☐ feeling irresponsible or immature, like I'm not taking care of myself.

☐ the alcoholic hangover. (Much more severe than the "normal hangover," it can last from 3 to 10 days. With DTs and convulsions, it becomes so serious it can kill.)

☐ getting angry too often.

☐ feeling guilty or ashamed because of something I did after drinking too much.

☐ lying about my drinking. I lie to others and even to myself.

☐   denying that I have any problems from excessive drinking (even denying some of the problems in this worksheet).

☐   feeling more stressed.

☐   destroying my ability to work well.

☐   being stuck in a struggle.

☐   feeling exhausted or worn out.

☐   messing up my sleep. (Too much alcohol disturbs sleep, especially REM, or dream, sleep.)

☐   having the shakes in the morning.

☐   staying addicted. The more I drink, the more I want to drink.

☐   feeling as if I have no choice. Alcohol takes my freedom away.

☐   Other alcohol-related problems I want to avoid:

_____

_____

_____

_____

_____

_____

_____

_____

_____

Alcohol causes these problems. But alcohol solves many of these problems as well—for instance, tension, anxiety, depression, feeling stressed, feeling lost or lonely, the morning shakes. How often do you use alcohol to solve the very problems it causes? Take another look at your Worksheet #2: Reasons for Drinking.

Alcohol solves some problems. But it makes the same problems get worse. That's what's called the vicious circle of addiction.

From this point of view, alcoholic drinking seems like a tremendous waste of time. Why bother? All you gain is bad health and an early death. But when you quit drinking, you break out of the vicious circle. And, for the first time in years, you give yourself a chance to grow.

A new you, a solid you, a more interesting, nonaddicted you begins to show itself. It gets stronger and stronger the longer you abstain from alcohol.

DO YOU WANT TO QUIT?

Now you can make a decision. It's a mighty task, weighing the benefits against the problems. But by this time, you have a good feel for it. What to do? Quit . . . or keep drinking? If you keep drinking, how long will you continue before you need to quit?

One thing for sure, if you keep drinking, you get fewer benefits and more problems. The life of an alcoholic drinker becomes nearly impossible. To get an idea, take a good look at some older alcoholics you know (or knew) and imagine yourself in their place.

It's up to you. You may decide to quit drinking now. Or you may decide to wait. Either way, Worksheet #4: Reasons for Quitting will help. Your other work in this chapter has been leading to this one important list. When you quit drinking, you'll use this list over and over again.

Worksheet # 4

Reasons for Quitting

Instructions: Any problems alcohol is causing become your best reasons for quitting. So first, take another look at Worksheet #3.

Now on this worksheet, instead of looking at the problems (the negative), you'll see what you stand to gain (the positive). For instance, instead of the problem "I'll die younger," here you'll note what happens when you quit drinking: "I'll live longer."

On this worksheet you'll see some good reasons for quitting. Check any you feel are important to you. Then in the blank lines, write your own reasons for quitting. To do this, review the problems you checked in Worksheet #3 and rewrite each problem to reflect a positive benefit you will gain when you quit.

☐ I'll live longer.

☐ I can greatly reduce my chances of getting cirrhosis.

☐ My liver will begin to heal.

☐ I'll be a more productive worker.

☐ I'll have more energy.

☐ I'll feel stronger at everything I do.

☐ I'll have better digestion.

☐ It will help me cut down on smoking.

☐ It will help me get things done more quickly.

☐ I'll feel more relaxed.

☐ I'll be able to think more clearly.

☐ I'll set a good example for my children.

☐ I'll have more time.

☐ I'll have more money.

☐ I'll feel happier.

☐ I'll feel liberated, free to do what I want.

☐ I'll get in control of my life.

- ☐ I'll gain self-confidence.
- ☐ I'll feel more mature.
- ☐ I'll feel like I've finally started making smart decisions.
- ☐ I'll regain my creativity.
- ☐ I'll become healthy . . . I won't feel as sick all the time.
- ☐ I'll have a better voice, a stronger, clearer throat.
- ☐ It will improve my nerves . . . I'll stop feeling nervous and tense.
- ☐ I'll be able to show my good qualities more often.
- ☐ I'll feel stronger emotionally.
- ☐ I can start healing. My body will repair most of the damage alcohol has done.
- ☐ I can reduce my high blood pressure.
- ☐ I can avoid pancreatitis.
- ☐ I can avoid _____ (any other serious health problem that concerns you).

Continue your reasons for quitting by rewriting problems from Worksheet #3:

_____

_____

_____

_____

_____

_____

_____

_____

Now do one last thing. Rank your reasons for quitting in order of importance to you. Just put a 1 in front of the reason that is most important to you, a 2 in front of the next most important reason, and so on.

What are your seven most important reasons? Write them here:

1. _____
2. _____
3. _____
4. _____
5. _____
6. _____
7. _____

I suggest you write these on a 3x5 file card and carry them with you everywhere. Review them whenever you feel you want a drink.

PART TWO

Planning Your Own Personal Approach to Quitting

CHAPTER 4

What About AA?

To be social is to be forgiving.
    —*Robert Frost*

Have friends. 'Tis a second existence.
    —*Baltasar Gracián y Morales*

A A offers social support based on a model of religious fellowship. Members help each other stay sober. At meetings members talk about their problems and gain guidance from each other. Each member also works through the "12 Steps." These steps give the recovering alcoholic a set of goals to be achieved. Some steps offer moral and ethical corrections to help you turn your life around. Other steps help you find peace in God or gain strength through God "as you understand Him."

AA has been helping alcoholics quit drinking since 1935. Current membership is about 1 million in the United States, about 2 million worldwide. AA is probably the most recommended treatment for alcoholics today. In fact, the format has become so popular that many look-alike programs have sprouted in the past 20 years. Some programs, using the same group methods and similar 12 steps include:

Alanon (for family members of alcoholics)

Alateen (for teenage family members of alcoholics)

Gamblers Anonymous

Narcotics Anonymous

ACOA (Adult Children of Alcoholics) groups

Overeaters Anonymous

Sex Addicts Anonymous

Indeed, AA can be a very successful method for quitting drinking. Unfortunately, its success seems highly limited. In the United States, only about 5% of alcoholic drinkers choose to use AA.

Of course, if AA is right for you, it can work wonders. This chapter will help you decide whether AA is for you; if it is, be sure to use AA as one of the key methods in your approach to quitting.

On the other hand, if you happen to be one of the 95% who don't feel comfortable with AA, or who don't like its methods, you needn't waste your time with it. In this book, you'll find many alternatives that will work for you.

HOW AA CAN HELP

AA can help you in many ways. In addition to those already mentioned, here are some other ways AA can help:

- It offers total involvement in a nonalcoholic community. This makes it easier for you to break away from your total involvement with alcohol. When you join AA, you join a ready-made social scene to replace the alcoholic social scene.

- As an AA member, you gain an important sense of belonging. When you belong to a valued organization, you feel more valued inside yourself.

- Group members lend mutual support for not drinking. This can be very helpful. As a popular song says, "We all need somebody to lean on."

- It's easy to make new friends in AA. You will have something in common with everyone you meet.

- AA destigmatizes alcoholism. You're not seen as a "disgusting drunk," but someone with a disease. More important, it's not your fault.

- AA helps you regain a sense of responsibility. You're not responsible for your disease, but you are responsible for maintaining your sobriety. It's up to you to stay away from alcohol. You'll find this new sense of responsibility will help you immensely.

- In any treatment, you first need to accept your problem with alcohol before you can begin to change. AA helps you accept your problem with alcohol. The method works well for many people. You start by admitting your problem in front of the group: "Hello. My name is _____, and I'm an alcoholic." Then in Step #1, you admit your problem to yourself.

- You can count on it. You can find meetings at many different times during the day, seven days a week. Also, once you've started, you're assigned a sponsor who's available 24 hours a day, seven days a week.

- It's free, or available for a small donation at each meeting. This could be very important to you. Other treatments can cost thousands of dollars,

and if you don't have health insurance you may
not be able to afford them.

Practice #2

Try a Few Meetings

Instructions: To discover whether AA is for you, try at
least five A A meetings. First, get a schedule of meetings
in your area. (You can have a schedule sent to you by call-
ing the local phone number for AA. Just look up Alcoholics Anonymous in your phone book.) Then select a few
meetings and begin going to them.

If you like the first meeting you go to, keep attending
that one. If you don't like it, shop around. Each AA group
has a personality all its own and it may take you a while
to find one you like.

Make notes if you want. It helps many people to write
about their experiences. You can write your ideas and your
feelings about AA in your notebook.

Important rule: Don't go drunk to the meetings. It's not
fair to anyone, especially yourself. If you don't have a
sober break in your drinking long enough to go to a meeting, wait until after you quit drinking, then do Practice #2.

DRAWBACKS TO AA

Many professionals and former AA members have
specific complaints about the organization's methods
and beliefs. Here's a list of the most common criti-
cisms:

- AA neglects the physical. You get no medical
  advice and no information on healing. You get

no encouragement to exercise, change your diet, learn relaxation or stress reduction techniques or any helpful methods—other than AA. In fact, you might think AA was encouraging *bad* health habits. At many meetings, sodas, cookies, cakes, or doughnuts are served; so are coffee and tea. Of course, both sugar and caffeine increase anxiety and nervous tension, especially in recovering alcoholics who have a heightened reaction to these substances. (Note: In recent years, some AA meetings have changed somewhat. Now you can find some meetings whose members are knowledgeable about health and serve only healthy foods and beverages. You can also find a few meetings that are non-smoking.) This is perhaps AA's biggest weakness. Even if you use AA, you'll do much better if you choose various other techniques to help you heal the physical problems alcohol has caused.

- AA requires social involvement. You gain help by becoming part of a group. But what if you're the type of person who gets nervous in groups? This can feel like a major punishment. Many people drink to help themselves in social situations, to feel calm around others. Yet AA forces you to be around others without the alcohol. Facing this prospect, you may get terribly nervous.

  I know many folks who tried AA, and as soon as the meeting was over headed straight for a bar. If group situations cause this kind of anxiety in you, you may find difficulty gaining any help from AA.

- AA requires a specific religious belief. You must believe in God or some greater power. Otherwise, you'll be lost. Six of the 12 steps refer to God or a greater power. In these six steps, you must turn yourself over to God, admit things to God, ask God for help, and seek God through prayer or meditation.

AA allows some flexibility in beliefs. God can be "as you understand Him." Even so, you may still have difficulty with a certain defined concept of God. For instance, you may not see God as a "Him."

Before quitting drinking, most alcoholics find that their strongest religious beliefs concern "God, the Bottle." Many have given up their faith in "God, the Father" long ago. If you can renew your belief in some kind of God when you quit the alcohol, AA may be of help. Otherwise, if you don't fit AA's religious format, don't worry. You can use any of the various spiritual religious alternatives mentioned later in this book.

• AA insists that you call yourself an alcoholic. You may be a lot of interesting things, but at every meeting—if you speak—you must start by saying, "Hello. My name is _____, and I'm an alcoholic." This reminds you, over and over, of a problem you have—not something good about you, but a problem. This negative reminder can help some people stay away from the problem (alcohol). But it forces some to feel too guilty too often, or to feel just plain stuck. At one meeting, you might like to hear everybody get up and say something positive like, "Hello. My name is _____, and I feel excited, happy, and refreshingly new today."

• Many folks have difficulty with the "public confessional" approach of AA. At meetings, members recount their problems with alcohol. This might be helpful if it didn't take so much time every meeting.

Stories about past problems have been called "drunkalogues." You'll hear details such as "the worst things I did while drunk," or "how bad a drunk I was," and so on. Too many of these stories makes for a mighty dreary meeting.

In addition, members complain about how difficult things are now that they're not drinking. You'll hear about "how much I wanted to drink today when the boss yelled at me," or "how terrible I have felt," or "how I've had a tough time fighting the urge to drink all day," and other similar complaints.

You might prefer more of an accent on the positive. Once again, if members dwelled more on the powerful, positive notes of their recovery, meetings could be much more uplifting.

- Some have accused AA of fostering too much dependency among its members. It's like trading one addiction for another, alcohol for AA. The new habit—going to meetings—beats the old habit in many ways. But some folks have difficulty giving so much of their lives to the group.

  After going to AA for a few months, one member said she felt "completely swallowed up by the group," as if she were losing her identity. This problem with AA will be greatest among independent-minded persons.

- For AA members, alcohol remains the central focus in their lives. Before AA, members were preoccupied with drinking. In AA, they're preoccupied with not drinking. Now instead of remembering the good old days, they remember how bad things were. Members recall problem after problem as they discuss the evils of alcohol.

That means they cannot break their relationship with alcohol. It's a love-hate relationship, but instead of leaving the relationship completely, they simply shift their involvement from love to hate.

- AA members believe you're powerless over alcohol. Is that true? It may be true before you quit. But don't you show some power over alcohol when you quit? Don't you show even greater and greater power over alcohol the longer you stay away from it?

- Members believe "Once an alcoholic, always an alcoholic." The idea is good. It tells you not to drink—or you'll become addicted all over again. So it helps you stay away from alcohol.

  But once you've decided you will not drink again, why not drop the idea that you're still an alcoholic? You don't call yourself a smoker after you've quit smoking, even though you know you'll be addicted if you start again. That's why the statement "Once an alcoholic, always an alcoholic" is not exactly true. A truer way to phrase it is this: "Once an alcoholic, always an alcoholic . . . *as long as you keep on drinking.*"

  If you believe you're an alcoholic forever—even when you're not drinking—you may feel stuck in a rut forever. What a grim outlook! The belief doesn't allow you any room to grow into something different.

  After you've quit drinking, you don't have to consider yourself an alcoholic. Think about this for a minute. If you change your diet, start exercising, and begin using other healing techniques, you can cure most of the disease problems alcohol has caused. You can keep growing, changing. You can be someone new and interesting every day, someone other than "an alcoholic."

- You may decide AA takes too much of your time. The hours you spend at AA every week you could be spending at some other positive or healthful activity.

IT'S YOUR CHOICE

You've gone to a few meetings. You know some of the good points about AA. You also know most of the reservations you have about it. So now you can make a decision.

Worksheet #5

My Decision About AA

Instructions: On the left side, write what you like about AA. On the right side, write what you don't like. Write each statement in your own words.

What I like about AA: *What I don't like about AA:*

_____   _____

_____   _____

_____   _____

_____   _____

What I like about AA:	*What I don't like about AA:*
_____	_____
_____	_____
_____	_____
_____	_____
_____	_____
_____	_____
_____	_____
_____	_____
_____	_____
_____	_____
_____	_____
_____	_____

Now evaluate your feelings and make a decision whether or not to join AA. (If you're still not sure, try a few more meetings.) Check one of the four boxes below:

☐ I like AA. I have no problems with it and I will use AA when I quit drinking.

☐ I like AA. The problems I have with it don't bother me that much, so I will use AA when I quit.

☐ I like some things about AA. But the problems I have with it bother me too much. I will not use AA when I quit.

☐ I don't like AA. I have too many problems with it. It will make things much harder for me, so I've decided not to use AA when I quit.

This is your decision. You can always change your mind later if you need to. No problem. But you've made up your mind for now. *So go with it.*

CHAPTER 5

How to Break a Habit

Habit, n. A shackle for the free.
        —Ambrose Bierce

Wise living consists perhaps less in acquiring good habits than in acquiring as few habits as possible.

        —Eric Hoffer

E verybody has habits, big habits, small habits. Some people have only a few habits. Some people have many.

In one sense, habits make life a little more convenient. Certain things seem easier. With just one way to do something, there's no need to think or to find a new way to do the same thing each time you approach it.

The problem is, you can get stuck in a rut. The more you do things by habit, the less adventure you have in your life, the less room for creativity. Too many habits or one very serious habit can chain you down. You can lose your sense of freedom. In fact, it can get to the point where you feel you're not doing anything new, just doing everything over and over by memory.

ALL ABOUT HABITS

What is a habit? A habit is a behavior you repeat again and again. Once you learn a behavior that helps you in some way, you tend to repeat it. Soon it becomes a normal behavior for you. After a few repetitions, it becomes habit.

Here's how a habit begins:

1. You find a certain way to do something.
2. It works. (It accomplishes your goal or it solves some problem for you.)
3. You stick to it. (You repeat the behavior over and over.)
4. You stop looking for other ways to do the same thing. (There may be many other ways to accomplish the same goal, but why look for them now?)

Habits develop for good reasons. You would not repeat the behavior otherwise. Even bad habits develop for good reasons. For instance, in Chapter 3 (Worksheet #2), you looked at some of the good reasons you have for drinking.

On the other hand, all habits cause some problems. Bad habits get worse, especially addictions. The longer you stay stuck in a bad habit, the more problems it causes. For instance, on Worksheet #3, you determined what personal problems alcohol causes. Even good habits cause problems. For example, you may develop the good habit of exercising. But when you must do the same workout the same way each day or else feel miserable, you lose some freedom. In a sense, you relinquish some control over a part of your life.

Of course, the good you gain from the habit of exercising far outweighs the drawbacks. But with a habit like alcoholism, the good you gain dwindles and the problems it causes begin to rule your entire life. Clearly, if you could simply exchange the habit of alcohol for the habit of exercise in your life, you'd be doing yourself a magnificent favor.

Back to Basics

A habit is something you do the *same way* each time you do it. The more you vary the way you do something, the less of a habit it is.

Furthermore, a habit is usually the *only way* you use to accomplish a certain goal.

Habits can be simple or complex. Complex habits come in two kinds. The first combines many simple habits. This kind of complex habit could be called a routine or a ritual. The second kind is based on a long-standing, deeply ingrained pattern of behavior. This kind of complex habit is the most difficult to break. Here are some examples:

Simple habits

putting on clothes in the same order all the time

combing your hair the same way all the time

brushing teeth

taking showers

shaving

putting on makeup

washing the dishes, mowing the lawn, or doing

some other household chore the same way
every time

sitting in the same chair for every meal or every
time you watch TV

Complex habits (combination of simple habits):

Morning ritual, a habitual way of handling all the
things you need to do each morning. For instance, you may get up at the same time each
workday, have coffee, take a shower, shave or
fix your hair, get dressed, have breakfast, brush
your teeth, and leave for work at about the
same time every day. You perform each of
these tasks in the same way and in the same
order each day.

Complex habits (long-standing, deeply ingrained):

Eating habits—not just the way you approach food
(for example: try eating with chopsticks, or
with your fork in the other hand), but the foods
you eat. Habits for certain foods run very deep.
That's why most people have great difficulty
changing their diets. Each of us tends to eat the
exact same foods week after week. And when
we don't eat these foods, we tend to eat the
same amounts of various types of ingredients.
This holds true right down to the amount of
salt, fat, protein, carbohydrates, and the total
number of calories we consume. Each person
has his or her own unique set of food addictions.

Personality. What we call personality is an
individual's *habitual* way of acting, a long-
standing pattern of behavior.

Posture. Holding your body in a certain way, carrying yourself in a certain way, usually favoring the same style over and over.

Sexual behavior. Sexual compulsions and other unique sexual behavior appear to be deeply ingrained habits. Excessive or unusual sexual behaviors have been called "sexual addictions."

Emotional behavior. Each person has a deeply ingrained pattern for dealing with stress. Most of us tend to use the same reaction every time we have a problem—and use this reaction instead of trying to solve each problem separately. A person's customary reaction could be anger, violence, crying, whining, complaining, becoming silent, and so on.

Addictions are the same as deeply ingrained complex habits, but they take only a short time to develop. You can become addicted to most substances in less than a year. Many addictions take less than two months to develop, and a few powerful drugs appear to addict the first or second time used.

Here are some examples of addictive substances:

caffeine

sugar (sugar addiction may be considered a very powerful food addiction, but withdrawal from it looks more like withdrawal from a drug)

nicotine

alcohol (actually two addictions rolled into one: sugar addiction plus sedative drug)

heroin and other opium-derived drugs (such as codeine, morphine)

cocaine (including "crack")

barbiturates, sedatives, tranquilizers

amphetamines

marijuana

Addictions change your biochemistry quickly and dramatically. That's why they become so strong and powerful. All your cells, especially your brain cells, crave the addictive substance. Without the substance, you start climbing the walls. You may feel nervous, depressed, sleepy, even a little crazy when you try to withdraw from the addictive substance.

To one degree or another, all habits are difficult to quit. Even breaking a simple habit takes care and concentration.

BREAKING HABITS, MAKING CHANGES

Here are five steps to help you break a habit. You need to:

1. Know you can change.
2. Unlearn learned behavior.
3. Make a decision to change.
4. Cope with cravings (or compulsions).
5. Find something to replace the habit.

If you follow these steps, you can break any habit. Now here's a detailed look at each step.

Step 1: Know You Can Change

When you know you can change, you can. Confidence is everything.

This seems like such a simple thing. But many people believe they can't change. They've convinced themselves of this. They believe that the way they are is the only way they can be. So, right from the start, they're stuck.

But this belief is just not true. Everybody can change. Anybody can change. You can too. You can change any habit if you put your mind to it.

Millions of very serious alcoholics have quit drinking. They found it hard. But they stayed with it and they were successful. You can be successful too.

As you learn what to do, you'll become more and more confident. So show your confidence. And show your strength. You can make no greater demonstration of strength in the world than by quitting a serious addiction.

Step 2: Unlearn Learned Behavior

Habits are learned. You learn that certain behaviors help you in certain ways. The more you think a behavior helps you, the more you tend to repeat it.

You may have the habit of crying (or complaining) because it helps you get your way. You may drink alcohol because it makes some of your problems seem easier to deal with. But remember: Any behavior that can be learned can be unlearned.

What does it mean to unlearn something? It means you find another way to accomplish the same goal. You find another behavior (instead of crying or complaining) to help you get your way. You learn other ways to cope with life's problems (instead of drinking).

Any habit can be changed. Some habits are easy to change, others more difficult. In Practice #3, you'll break a few habits. When you do this, you'll see what it takes to unlearn a habit.

Meanwhile, if you haven't already quit drinking, start considering how you'll break the drinking habit. Whenever you drink, remind yourself that you'd rather not be an alcoholic for the rest of your life. Drinking doesn't fit in with your long-range plans. You're going to change. You're going to learn something new. You don't want to continue drinking excessively. Soon you'll quit completely! Remind yourself you'd rather have better health, be slimmer, trimmer, look better, feel better, live longer, think more clearly, deal with your problems more maturely, and finally feel liberated.

During the next few weeks, think of ways to deal with your problems *without drinking*. And think of things you could be doing instead of drinking. For instance, what things would you like to do if drinking didn't take so much of your time? What things do you miss when you drink too much?

For the next few weeks, whenever you drink, think of the things you miss. Later in this chapter, you can list them in Checklist #2.

Step 3: Make a Decision to Change

How do you make a decision to change? Keep three points in mind. You must:

- *Want to change.* This means your heart is in it. The more you want to do something, the stronger your decision will be to do it.

- *Take responsibility for yourself.* Take responsibility for any problems that you cause through your habit. When you take responsibility for what you do, you can break a habit. (Remember too: Take responsibility for any new behavior that replaces your habit. It gives you a chance to feel proud.)

- *Have a clear goal or a clear set of goals.* For instance, when quitting drinking, most people have two main goals: getting themselves free and regaining good health.

With these three points, you can turn your decision to quit drinking into a lifelong commitment and your sobriety into a welcomed joy.

Step 4: Cope with Cravings (or Compulsions)

A habit is something you feel compelled to do. Even when you quit it, you still feel compelled to do it. If it's a habit related to food, drugs, or alcohol, you have cravings when you quit. If it's a habit related to a behavior, you have compulsions to repeat the behavior.

Addictions consist of cravings and compulsions. When you quit, you crave the addictive substance and feel compelled to use it again. For a while after you quit, your cravings and compulsions get stronger. Why? Your body wants to re-create the addiction-induced equilibrium. Over time, your cravings and compulsions diminish as your body adjusts to a new equilibrium.

To quit any addiction successfully, you need to cope with your cravings and compulsions. Probably the single best way to cope is simply to wait them out. How do you do this? Each time you have a craving or compulsion, don't act on it, but simply be aware of it. Watch how it operates in your mind. And wait. While you watch and wait, your relaxed awareness will free you from the craving in a short amount of time.

What can you do during this period of time? Try continuing whatever activity you were involved in. Or try deep breathing. Try exercise. Try any of the relaxation techniques in this book. Drink water, fruit juice, club soda, or herb tea. Eat a healthy snack, such as carrot or celery sticks, popcorn, nuts, fruit, dried fruit (raisins, prunes), corn chips, rice cakes, and so on. Try doing any of your alternatives to drinking (see Checklist #2, next section).

When you first quit drinking, cravings are very strong. That means you need to be just as strong to deal with them. But don't worry—you can do it. In this book, you'll learn many techniques that will work for you. Just be sure to use them.

And remember: The longer you stay away from alcohol, the easier it gets. Coping with your cravings does get easier. The main reason? You get stronger and stronger.

Step 5: Find Something to Replace the Habit

A habit helps you do a certain thing in a certain way. When you quit the habit, immediately you feel something is missing. You find yourself with an empty space of time.

You can fill this time in two ways:

1. You can find a new way to do the same thing.
2. You can do something completely different.

Let's look at these options.

1. Find a new way to do the same thing: For instance, you may brush your teeth a certain way every time. When you break the habit, you can find a new way to clean your teeth. You can concentrate on a new method of brushing, change your pattern of brushing, or find some other method that doesn't include brushing, such as flossing with baking soda and rinsing with salt water.

What about the drinking habit? Alcohol helps you get high. When you quit it, you could find other drugs that will get you high. But then you get addicted to these drugs. The solution? Find other (nondrug) ways to get high. Exercise works wonders. It's a different kind of high that creates a feeling of exhilaration. Relaxation techniques work, too. Even changing to a healthy diet helps you get high, as you gradually regain the glow of good health.

There's another way to look at it. The drinking habit helps you do many different things (see Worksheet #2.) When you quit drinking, you can find new ways to do any of these important things. You can find new ways to calm down, new ways to socialize, new ways to have fun, new ways to cope with certain problems.

Or you can . . .

2. Do something completely different: When you break a habit, you can use the time to do something else. If you choose this option, you abandon the habit as well as the goal of the habit.

When you quit drinking, you give up the goal of the habit: getting high or drunk. And you gain hours and hours of extra time. In fact, you gain so much extra time, this can become a problem in itself. You may feel as if you have too much time on your hands.

So when you quit drinking, you want to occupy yourself with other things you like to do. The more the better. Choose things you now miss because of your drinking.

Maybe you'd like fishing . . . or building models . . . or drawing . . . or writing . . . or doing anything artistic . . . or remodeling your home . . . or doing something enjoyable with your kids . . . or taking a class . . .

Soon after quitting drinking, you will find many

new ways to enjoy yourself. But for now, practice breaking a few habits and see how you do.

Practice #3

Pick a Few Habits and Break Them

Instructions: Pick a few of your habits and break them. Use the list below to make your selections.

Here you'll learn to break habits and gain the confidence that you can change your life. For simple habits and routines, you will learn to change the pattern of your behavior. For stronger habits and addictions, you will eliminate the behavior completely.

When breaking a habit, pay close attention to what happens inside of you. Notice your consciousness. If you don't remain conscious of what you're doing, even for a brief moment, you tend to slip and fall back into the same pattern. So stay alert. Notice also what works for you when dealing with cravings and compulsions. Make notes. Make sure you remember what techniques work best. You will use the same techniques to deal with cravings and compulsions when you quit drinking.

For this practice, pick one habit from the first group, one from the second, and one or two from the third group. Plan to break each habit for at least three weeks.

Simple Habits

Pick one of these habits and break it.

☐   Putting on shoes and socks. If you normally put on right sock, right shoe first, try putting on left sock, left shoe first.

☐   Taking a shower. If you normally wash your hair first and work your way down, try washing your feet first and work your way up. If you normally take a shower, start to take a bath instead.

- [ ] Shaving. Use a pattern different from the one you normally use.
- [ ] Combing hair. Comb your hair in a different way or in a different style every day.
- [ ] Cosmetics. Put your eye makeup on in a different way.
- [ ] Cracks in the sidewalk. If you normally avoid cracks in the sidewalk, start stepping on them.
- [ ] (Your idea) _____

Routines

Pick one and break it.

- [ ] Morning ritual. Do everything in a different order. Remember, you'll probably have to get up earlier. Or just do something *completely different*. Idea: Get up, run around the house a dozen times, come in through an open window, kiss everyone in the house three times each, write a few lines of poetry, then leave for work (oops . . . are you still in your pajamas?).
- [ ] Work routine. As much as possible, change your usual pattern. (Notice how your creativity at work begins to rise.)
- [ ] Evening ritual. Again, change the entire pattern as much as possible.
- [ ] Exercise routine.
- [ ] Watching TV. This is a very strong habit; some call it an addiction. Try quitting completely. Do you feel freer? What can you do with all that free time?
- [ ] (Your idea) _____

Stronger Habits and Addictions

You'll find these much more difficult to break, and therefore better practice for quitting drinking. Pick one or two and break each for three weeks at a time. Note: You may try recommended substitutes to help reduce cravings.

☐ Red meat, chicken, and eggs. (Try substituting fish or bean dishes.)

☐ Sugars. Many names: white sugar, brown sugar, molasses, honey, maple syrup, corn syrup, sucrose, glucose, dextrose, maltose, fructose. Very difficult to quit. Be aware of labels: Sugar is added to almost everything, even most brands of normal table salt. (To deal with craving, avoid chemical substitutes such as artificial sweeteners. Try fresh or dried fruit instead.)

☐ Dairy products: milk, butter, cheese, yogurt. (When doing this, eat lots of dark green vegetables like broccoli, kale, collards, and parsley. To satisfy craving, try eating seeds and nuts, especially sesame seeds, sesame butter, peanut butter, and almond butter. The dark leafy greens are high in calcium. So are sesame seeds and nuts.)

☐ White flour and white flour products. (Substitute whole grain flours such as whole wheat, whole oat, or rye. Read labels, but be careful: if it says "wheat flour," read "white flour"; it must say "100% whole wheat flour" or "100% stoneground whole wheat.")

☐ Foods with chemical preservatives and artificial flavors. (Another tough one. Read labels. Even fresh fruits and vegetables are chemically sprayed or treated, unless they say "organic" or "organically grown.")

☐ Caffeine. Includes coffee, regular teas, cocoa, chocolate, some headache medicines, and many types of soda.

☐ Nicotine. Includes all tobacco products. This is a major addiction. If you can quit smoking, you can quit drinking.

☐ Quit any other drug you take regularly. Pick one: marijuana, diet pills, cocaine, uppers or downers, or even an over-the-counter drug such as a headache remedy, a nasal spray, or cough suppressant. (*Important note*: Don't quit any prescribed medication without doctor's orders.)

☐ (Your idea:) _____

WHAT ELSE CAN YOU DO?

Jump. Excite yourself. Ignite your mind with wonder, awe, enchantment. Fill yourself to the brim with lust for life. Utter unusual sounds. Envision waterfalls. Spin with vibrant pulsing energy. Reel . . . and rock . . . and roll.

Sit cross-legged on the table. Do somersaults on the ground. Smile. Laugh out loud.

Do it all without alcohol.

Some people ask, "When I quit drinking, what else can I do?" You can do a hundred different things. Two hundred different things. Anything you choose.

When you quit drinking, you open a whole new world. Instantly, you gain a great amount of time. At first you may be surprised at how much extra time you have.

Why does this happen? As an alcoholic drinker, you spend so much of your life preoccupied with alcohol. When you make plans, you make sure to include alcohol in them. Sometimes you don't make any plans except for the alcohol—you just know, whatever you do, you're going to drink. Sometimes when it's just you and the booze, you may feel alcohol is your only friend.

By quitting drinking, you give yourself a great opportunity to do some different things—things you may miss doing now. With the extra time you gain, you can find many new and interesting ways to enjoy life, to overcome problems and to realize goals.

So it is important to make sure you find some new things to do, or new ways to enjoy the things you do already, when you quit. The more alternatives you have to drinking, the more exciting your life becomes.

In addition, your alternatives help you cope with cravings. They can help you cope with an immediate craving or help you when you're feeling tense. Some alternatives that take more time can seem like a total adventure away from alcohol.

An alternative for you may be something as simple as doodling on a piece of paper for a few minutes. Or it may be as complex as planning—and then going on—a special vacation. (By the way, when you quit drinking, you can save enough money in one year to afford a really fine vacation.)

So just remember, whenever you feel a craving for a drink, do one of your favorite alternatives. Quickly, you'll forget about the craving.

What are your favorite alternatives to drinking? Do Checklist #2 and find out.

Checklist #2

Alternatives to Drinking

Instructions: Which alternatives would you enjoy doing? Look these over and put a check next to any one you'd like to do. You can also write your own choices at the end of each category. (Keep in mind that if you associate any of these too much with drinking, if it's something you do while drinking, it might not be a good alternative for you when you quit.)

Now go back and pick your favorites. Put a second check next to any alternative you'd *really* like to do.

When you quit drinking, any one of your alternatives gives you a new way of enjoying life. But do your favorite ones first. It'll be more of a treat.

One other thing: Do not start doing any of these until after you quit drinking. In that way, you can use them as a reward for quitting.

Creative Hobbies and Crafts

- [ ] drawing
- [ ] writing
- [ ] sculpting
- [ ] painting
- [ ] music
- [ ] photography
- [ ] finger painting
- [ ] doodling
- [ ] collecting (anything from bottles to baseball cards, whatever suits your fancy)
- [ ] building models
- [ ] sewing/needlecraft
- [ ] knitting/crochet/tatting
- [ ] macramé/weaving
- [ ] ceramics
- [ ] model railroading
- [ ] woodworking/cabinetmaking
- [ ] tole painting/decoupage
- [ ] tie-dying
- [ ] metalwork/tinsmithing
- [ ] leatherwork
- [ ] making jewelry

Physical Activities

Exercise

- [ ] walking/hiking
- [ ] jogging/running
- [ ] hatha yoga/stretching exercises
- [ ] tai chi/karate
- [ ] swimming

- ☐ rowing/rowing machine
- ☐ canoeing/kayaking
- ☐ bicycling/bicycle machine
- ☐ snow skiing/water skiing/skiing machine
- ☐ surfing/windsurfing
- ☐ trampoline
- ☐ dancing
- ☐ aerobic exercise classes
- ☐ roller skating
- ☐ ice skating
- ☐ weight lifting/weight lifting and conditioning machines
- ☐ jumping rope
- ☐ any exercise routine or workout

Sport

- ☐ any above exercise or training, if done competitively:

_____

_____

- ☐ tennis/badminton
- ☐ racquetball/handball/squash
- ☐ baseball/softball
- ☐ volleyball
- ☐ basketball
- ☐ soccer
- ☐ field hockey/ice hockey
- ☐ golf
- ☐ bowling
- ☐ boating
- ☐ fishing
- ☐ croquet/bocci

Home and Garden Projects

☐ any home fix-it or repair job
☐ auto repair work
☐ mowing the lawn
☐ installing a fence
☐ cooking a new recipe
☐ planting flower beds, trees, shrubbery
☐ installing a rock garden, sidewalk, patio
☐ any home improvement (painting, redecorating, re-modeling)
☐ gardening (a lot of work with a clear benefit: raising good food for your table)
☐ farming ("large-scale" gardening—may include raising animals)

Intellectual Pursuits

☐ teaching yourself something new
☐ taking classes
☐ getting a degree
☐ reading a book
☐ going to a museum
☐ making plans to do something special.
☐ working on your own personal life-plans (this book gives you ideas on making new plans for a changing life)
☐ studying something you'd like to know more about—what interests you: _____
☐ teaching somebody something you've learned

Spiritual Pursuits

☐ religious activity (church, religious events)
☐ studying spiritual teachings
☐ practicing meditation or prayer

☐ taking time for self-reflection

☐ working with any spiritual techniques to gain personal inspiration and enlightenment

☐ working AA's 12 Steps (the spiritual and moral backbone of AA.)

☐ taking a spiritual self-help workshop

☐ reviewing your morality—determining what's right and wrong for you—and following it

Social/Emotional Activities

Helping Yourself

☐ spending more time with friends

☐ spending more time with loved ones

☐ improving the quality of your friendships

☐ improving your loving relationships (may try: ☐ workshops, ☐ marriage counseling, ☐ family therapy)

☐ working on getting rid of emotional problems (may try: ☐ self-study with books, ☐ workshops, ☐ counseling or individual therapy, ☐ group therapy)

☐ learning stress reduction and relaxation techniques

☐ learning assertiveness (how to stick up for yourself without being too aggressive)

☐ finding one new nondrinking friend

☐ developing a whole new set of friends

Helping Others

☐ doing something special for somebody else

☐ getting yourself on a program to do one kind thing for someone every day

☐ doing volunteer work at hospitals or for local service organizations

☐ being a Scout leader

☐ being more helpful to others at work

- [ ] joining Alcoholics Anonymous, Women for Sobriety, Rational Recovery, or Secular Organizations for Sobriety (in these groups, you help others overcome their problems with alcohol)
- [ ] becoming a Big Brother/Big Sister
- [ ] visiting an elderly relative or friend
- [ ] giving to a charity or join a charity group

Vacations, Games, and Entertainment

- [ ] getting away from it all: a vacation, special trip, or family outing
- [ ] visiting a recreation center
- [ ] going to an amusement park
- [ ] special events: concerts, sporting events
- [ ] going out to dinner
- [ ] going to a movie
- [ ] playing a game with family or friends: card games, board games, any kind of game
- [ ] playing solitaire (if you can make it a lively enough game!)
- [ ] working a crossword puzzle or any kind of puzzle
- [ ] listening to music
- [ ] reading a book or magazine
- [ ] pampering yourself (your choice):
  - [ ] a hot bath or long shower
  - [ ] a visit to the beauty salon
  - [ ] a shave at a barbershop
  - [ ] cooking a meal you really like
  - [ ] buying yourself a gift

Work

☐   getting better at your work (this will come naturally;
     when you quit drinking, you will have more energy
     for your work)

☐   starting a new business (choose something you can do
     very well)

YES, YOU CAN CHANGE

If you want to change something about yourself, how
do you do it? What's the best way?

First, you need to know what part of you you want
to change. You need to understand it completely.
Then, when you understand it completely, you can
drop it completely. You can let the whole thing go.

With alcoholism, you need to understand the
whole picture. What makes you want to drink? Why
do you drink too much? How does it affect you? You
need to know the benefits you get from drinking as
well as the problems it causes. Then, when you quit
drinking, you can drop the whole behavior—the benefits and the problems. Soon you will find new ways to
get the same benefits. And of course, you will enjoy
getting rid of the problems.

Here's another way to visualize a major change in
your life, such as quitting drinking: View the "alcoholic self" as a whole separate part of you you no
longer want. Then, when you're ready to change, kill
the old alcoholic self. Now watch a new self emerge,
a new, interesting nonalcoholic self. It's like being
born anew.

Many people who have quit their alcoholism look
back at the time they quit as a time of rebirth, a time
of total transformation. The butterfly emerges from
its chrysalis, never to be a caterpillar again.

It's Your Decision

Look in the mirror. Is that the same person you saw in the mirror yesterday? Is it the same person you saw there a year ago?

You continue to change whether you like it or not. Every day you change. You are not the same "you" you were yesterday. Some of the cells that were "you" yesterday are dead and gone. New cells have taken their place.

You are not even the same person you were five minutes ago. Things change. You are continually becoming someone new, someone different from who you were before.

How can it help you to know this?

It helps to free you. It helps you realize that you're not stuck. And when you are not stuck, that means you are free to change.

You keep changing anyway. No matter what, you continue to change. You can change for the better or you can change for the worse.

It's up to you.

CHAPTER 6

Healing Through Diet

*One cannot think well, love well, sleep well
if one has not dined well.*
                    —*Virginia Woolf*

*It's a very odd thing—
As odd as can be—
That whatever Miss T. eats
Turns into Miss T.*
                    — *Walter de la Mare*

W ithout a doubt, diet is the single most important component of good health. It's miraculous
how much healing takes place when you change from
a poor diet to a healthy one. Think about it. Whatever
you eat and drink becomes an intimate part of you.
You swallow your food and immediately your body
begins to assimilate it. Through digestion, you become one with what you eat and drink. Through digestion your body gains important nutrients.

The nutrients in food form the building blocks of
life itself. You gain strength from food. The strength
of every cell in your body depends on the quality of

the food you eat. How can you enjoy high-quality health? Eat high-quality foods.

Another benefit: Your mental and emotional health will improve. Through good nutrition, you can dramatically enhance your brain's biochemical functioning. A balanced diet will make you feel balanced and energized. Such a diet enables you to think clearly, act calmly, and deal effectively with stress.

When you quit drinking, you can do yourself a big favor by changing your diet. A good diet can improve your emotional outlook and heal most of the physical damage caused by excessive drinking.

The process is gradual but amazing. As you get healthier, you begin to feel younger. You even begin to look younger. You have more zest. This goes on for many years after you quit drinking. It's as if you have added lost years back onto your life.

What's more, the better the diet, the more effective the healing. It may take you a while to learn how to follow a healthy diet, but the effort is definitely worth it.

THE IMPORTANCE OF DIET

Consider your diet. Are you getting the nutrients you need? If you drink excessively, the answer is no.

When you drink more than a few drinks a week, you begin to have problems. Why? Alcohol reduces your body's ability to absorb nutrients. Too much alcohol in the diet causes malnutrition.

In addition, alcohol converts almost instantly to sugar. Over time you become hypoglycemic. This puts severe stresses on the liver, pancreas, adrenal glands, brain, and nervous system.

Furthermore, through continued excessive drinking, your alcohol metabolism continues to malfunction and your body takes longer to detoxify. Your liver, kidneys, and intestines get weaker. Meanwhile, as these organs break down, your addiction gets worse.

But when you quit drinking, you can change your biochemistry through diet. With a healthy diet, you can improve your body's nutrition, strengthen your metabolism, curb your cravings for alcohol, and become strong and healthy again.

A MATTER OF BALANCE

Your body seeks natural ways to balance itself. When out of balance, it craves whatever it needs to regain balance. That's why you crave certain foods at certain times. This applies to alcohol as well. Some of your craving for alcohol is due to your body's need to achieve internal balance.

Your body balances your food intake on two scales: contractive/expansive and acid/alkaline. Too contracted, the body will crave expansive foods. For instance, if you eat too many meats (extremely contractive), your body will crave sweets, or alcohol, or aspirin (extremely expansive). If you eat too many sweets or drink too much alcohol, you will crave meats, or eggs, or salty foods. Therefore, when you quit an extremely expansive food such as sugar or alcohol, you will find it easier to quit some of the extremely contractive foods in your diet as well.

On the other scale, if you have an internal acid condition, you'll crave alkaline foods. For instance, people tend to put lots of salt (alkalizing) on meat or eggs (acid-forming). People tend to like something sweet (acid-forming) with coffee (alkalizing). Vegetables (alkaline) balance grains, beans, or meat (acid-forming).

These "natural cravings" help you eat the right foods to keep you balanced—not necessarily healthy, but balanced. The body begins having problems when you you eat too many extreme foods. Like a pendulum, you swing from one extreme to another, making it almost impossible to stay in balance. It's like trying to balance a seesaw by stacking heavy rocks on each end when, really, all you have to do is stand in the middle.

Contractive/Expansive

Foods can be contractive or expansive. Basically, expansive foods open you up, contractive foods block you up. The body functions best in a mildly expanded state, slightly open. Thoughts come freely, blood flows freely, and the body eliminates waste easily.

When you eat too many contractive foods, you feel uptight, hard-headed, and possibly paranoid. Examples:

Extremely contractive foods

salt
red meat (beef, pork, lamb, veal)
eggs

Moderately contractive foods

chicken and other fowl
hard cheeses

Mildly contractive foods

fish

sea vegetables (kelp, Irish moss, dulse, wakame, hiziki, nori, agar)

Other foods cause you to feel expansive. If you consume too many of these foods, you get spaced-out, confused, and possibly out of control. Examples:

Extremely expansive foods

drugs and medications
alcohol
vinegar
sugar (all types, including honey and maple syrup)

Moderately expansive foods

fruit
dairy food (milk, soft cheeses, yogurt, butter)
nightshades (potatoes, tomatoes, eggplant, green pepper, red pepper, chili pepper, sweet peppers, paprika, cayenne)
most herbs and spices

Mildly expansive foods

vegetables (most varieties except nightshades)
seeds and nuts
beans

Some foods are almost evenly balanced for expansive and contractive qualities. These are centered foods. They help you remain centered. Examples:

whole wheat
brown rice
whole oats/oatmeal

barley
whole rye
corn/cornmeal
millet
buckwheat

Acid/Alkaline

Strong blood is mildly alkaline. The alkaline blood is strong because viruses and other bacteria cannot live in it.

Most people in America, however, have acidic blood, due to a diet high in acid-forming foods (meats and sweets, primarily). Examples:

Acid-forming foods (from most contractive to most expansive)

meat (including chicken and fish)
eggs
whole grains
beans (dried, cooked)
refined grains (white flour, white rice)
seeds and nuts
oil
sugar (all types, including honey and maple syrup)

Alkalizing foods (from most contractive to most expansive):

salt
fresh beans
sea vegetables

vegetables
nightshades
fruits
fruit juice
coffee

*Buffers—partly alkalizing, partly acid-forming
(from most contractive to most expansive):*

soy sauce and miso (fermented soybean products)
tofu (high-protein soy food)
cheeses
butter
milk

Finding Balance

It's fairly easy to balance your diet on the acid/alkaline and the expansive/contractive scales. Simply stop eating too many extreme foods.

Cut out meats and sweets, cut out alcohol and drugs, including nicotine. Cut out or cut back on coffee. Cut back on salt. Cut back on oils; cut out high-cholesterol fats and oils. Cut out eggs. Cut out or cut back on dairy foods. Cut out soft drinks. Cut out or cut back on any refined, processed, or partial foods, such as white flour (breads, pastas, pastries, desserts), white rice, lunch meats, and any products with sugars, chemicals, or preservatives added.

Increase the amount of whole grains, beans, vegetables, fruits, fish, seeds, and nuts. Sound familiar? This diet has been shown in study after study to be the best for maintaining optimum health. This is the diet recommended to decrease the risk of cancer. It's the same diet recommended to reduce cholesterol and the risk of heart disease. This diet will bring high blood pressure into normal ranges. This diet alleviates arthritis. This diet will control, and possibly cure, hypoglycemia. It will heal, and possibly cure, most of the ailments caused by alcoholism (see Checklist #1: Checklist of Medical Problems).

In short, the centered diet—as outlined on the next few pages—offers you the quickest, most complete way to heal yourself. Try it and see.

RECOMMENDED FOODS AND BEVERAGES

Whole Grains

Highly recommended; one of the most balanced foods you can eat. The body's natural digestion slowly breaks down the complex carbohydrates of whole grains into simple carbohydrates, food for the cells. This slow process gives the body steady energy for a few hours.

Eat cooked whole grains as much as possible. Gram for gram, you'll gain the most energy from these. Otherwise, eat ground whole grains in bread, crackers, pancakes, and rolls—or even occasional desserts made with barley malt or rice syrup instead of sugar. You can also eat whole grain in the form of rice cakes, popcorn, puffed wheat.

Whole grains should comprise 45% to 65% of your diet. Eat them as the main course for nearly every meal.

brown rice (short, medium, and long grain, basmati rice, sweet rice, and other varieties; also prepared in rice cakes) barley (pearl barley)

millet

whole oats (steel-cut oats, rolled oats, oatmeal;
     also roasted rolled oats in unsweetened or
     barley-malt sweetened granolas)

whole wheat (cracked wheat, bulgur; also 100%
     whole wheat bread, whole wheat noodles and
     pastas, puffed wheat, whole wheat pastries and
     desserts)

corn (corn grits, cornmeal, polenta; also cornbread,
     corn chips, tortillas, popcorn)

rye (whole rye; also whole grain rye breads and
     100% rye crackers)

buckwheat (buckwheat groats, kasha; also buck-
     wheat noodles and buckwheat flour for pan-
     cakes)

Beans

Highly recommended. A fairly balanced food, slightly
expansive, high in protein. Beans, when combined
with whole grains, offer a complete source of balanced
protein.

As you decrease the amount of meat in your diet,
you need to increase the amount of beans. But eat
small portions compared to the whole grains in your
meal.

Beans should form 5% to 20% of your diet. Eat
small portions once or twice a day.

chickpeas (garbanzos)

lentils

adzuki

black soybeans

black turtle beans

kidney beans

pinto beans

split peas (green or yellow)

navy beans

great northern beans

lima beans (dried)

red beans

black-eyed peas

bean products (such as tofu, tempeh, soy milk, soy condiments such as soy sauce and miso, various "natural burger" mixes using ground whole beans or peas)

Vegetables

Highly recommended. Fairly balanced, slightly expansive. Vegetables provide one of the best sources of vitamins and minerals to revitalize the body. What's more, the vitamins and minerals in vegetables are easy for the body to assimilate.

Vegetables should make up 20% to 30% of your diet, three to five servings a day. Of your vegetable intake, about 50% should come from green leafy vegetables, about 25% from root vegetables, and about 25% from squashes and other above-ground vegetables.

Dark green leafy

collard greens

kale

mustard greens

broccoli

parsley

scallions
watercress
dandelion greens
chicory
leeks
turnip greens
carrot greens
daikon and other radish greens
chives

Roots
carrots
onions
radishes
turnips
rutabagas
burdock
lotus root
parsnips

Above ground
squashes (acorn, butternut, pumpkin, Hubbard,
    pattypan, yellow/summer)
cabbage
brussels sprouts
Chinese cabbage
bok choy
cauliflower
mushrooms

shiitake mushrooms
celery
cucumbers
green peas
string beans (green, yellow/wax, purple, and others)
escarole
lettuce (head, Bibb, endive)
sprouts (grain, bean, alfalfa)
Sweet potatoes/yams (seek locally grown varieties)

Sea Vegetables

Highly recommended. Well balanced, slightly contractive. High in minerals, sea vegetables help the
body build strength and stamina. This is an important
food to help you balance your diet when cutting back
on meat. It should make up about 5% of your diet. Eat
small portions, maybe four or five times per week.

wakame (alaria)
dulse
Irish moss
hiziki
arame
kombu
nori
agar (kanten)

Seeds and Nuts

Recommended in small quantities. Fairly balanced,
moderately expansive. Both seeds and nuts contain
great amounts of protein and natural oils. Sesame

seeds are extremely high in calcium. Almonds are a good source of calcium as well. Eat small portions. Very good roasted.

Seeds

sesame

pumpkin

sunflower

Nuts

almonds

chestnuts

walnuts

peanuts

pecans

filberts

Brazil, hazel, cashew, pistachio (generally avoid these unless you live in a tropical climate)

Seed and Nut Butters

sesame butter, tahini

almond butter

peanut butter

sunflower butter

Fish and Fowl

Recommended for occasional use. Fairly balanced, slightly to moderately contractive. In small quantities, fish and fowl can be highly energizing. Both are high in protein, yet lower in fat than red meats. They

should make up about 5% of your diet. Eat in one or
two meals a week.

Fish/Seafood

bass
carp
cod
flounder
haddock
halibut
perch
salmon
scrod
sole
trout
turbot
whitefish
clams
mussels
oysters
scallops
tuna (somewhat unbalanced; use only once or
   twice a year, if at all)

Fowl

chicken
Cornish hens
duck
goose
turkey

Fruits

Recommended. Fairly balanced in small amounts. From moderately expansive for northern-grown fruits to extremely expansive for tropical fruits. Fruit helps clear the mind and open the body. But if you eat too much fruit, you can feel spaced out.

Fruit juice lacks the fiber of whole fruit and is recommended only in very small quantities (one or two ounces a day). Too much fruit juice can seriously weaken the intestines.

The rule of thumb for fruit is to eat whatever grows locally (within 200 miles of you) and eat it only when it is fresh and in season. If you live in the north, don't eat tropical fruit. In the north, local fresh fruit is not available through the winter, except for apples. Dried fruits such as raisins store well and can be eaten anytime.

Northern fruit (temperate zone)

apples

apricots

blackberries

blueberries

boysenberries

currants

cantaloupe

cherries

grapes (raisins)

honeydew melon

nectarines

peaches

pears

plums (prunes)
raspberries
strawberries
watermelon

Tropical fruit
lemons
persimmons
tangerines
avocados
bananas
coconuts
dates
figs
grapefruit
mangos
oranges
papayas
pineapples
pomegranates

Milk and Milk Products (Dairy Foods)

Not recommended. Fairly unbalanced. Moderately contractive (hard, salty cheeses), or moderately expansive (soft cheeses, milk, butter, yogurt, and cream).

These foods are high in calcium, but also high in phosphorus, which blocks the body's ability to assimilate calcium. You'll gain much better calcium absorption from dark green leafy vegetables.

Dairy foods are high in protein, yet also high in

cholesterol-type fats. Some dairy products now available have reduced fat: skim milk, 1% and 2% milk, and low-fat cheeses. These refined dairy foods should generally be avoided, however. They have been manufactured by removing the butterfat from whole milk. Without the butterfat, the assimilation of calcium decreases. Further, without the protein-splitting enzymes in butterfat, digestion of low-fat dairy foods becomes labored and incomplete. You will experience better digestion and better calcium absorption with the whole-milk alternatives.

Two-thirds of all people are allergic to dairy food. You may want to get tested to see whether you're one of them.

It's recommended to completely remove dairy foods from your diet, or to cut back considerably. One method to cut back: Quit all dairy foods for five or six days at a time, allowing yourself to have them only a day or two each week.

milk
butter
cheese
yogurt
cream
buttermilk
sour cream
ice cream (not recommended)
goat's milk and goat's milk products

Nightshade Vegetables

Not recommended. Fairly unbalanced, moderately expansive. Nightshade vegetables upset the body's calcium metabolism by causing a biochemical reaction that removes calcium from the bones and redeposits it, via the bloodstream, throughout the body. This causes inappropriate calcification in the joints, kidneys, blood vessels, and soft tissue, including brain tissue. Indeed, some specialists recommend eliminating the nightshades if you have any inappropriate calcification in the body, especially arthritis, osteoporosis, or other bone disease.

Interestingly, most diets high in nightshades will also be high in dairy foods. Most likely, the dairy foods offset at least some of the calcium loss from the nightshades.

For this reason, consider quitting dairy foods and nightshades together. Quitting only one at a time may cause calcium imbalances.

tomatoes

potatoes

eggplant

peppers (green, red, sweet, hot, bell, chili, paprika, cayenne)

tobacco (chewed or smoked, it causes imbalances as well)

Eggs

Not recommended. Unbalanced, very contractive. Eggs are high in protein but also very high in fat, especially cholesterol. It's a powerful, highly concentrated food. Eat only one a month, or none at all.

Oils

Recommended in small quantities for cooking or salad dressings. Fairly unbalanced, expansive. Unprocessed, unsaturated vegetable or seed oils can complement various foods and help with digestion. The following are recommended:

> unrefined dark sesame oil
>
> unrefined light sesame oil
>
> extra virgin olive oil
>
> pure expeller pressed safflower oil
>
> unrefined canola oil (should not be used for cooking)
>
> pure expeller pressed flaxseed oil (should not be used for cooking)

Natural Sweeteners

Recommended in small quantities if you crave sweets. Fairly unbalanced, expansive.

> barley malt
>
> rice syrup (yinnie syrup)
>
> juices (apple and other juices can be used as natural sweeteners in cooking)
>
> molasses
>
> maple syrup (in very small quantities)

Seasonings in Cooking

You can vary the flavor of foods by using different seasonings. You can vary the texture, the saltiness, the sweet and the sour, or add variety with herbs and spices.

> *Thickeners*
>
> kuzu
>
> arrowroot (powder or flour)
>
> agar (kanten)

For salty flavor

sea salt

miso (fermented soy paste: very good for making soups or sauces; many varieties, each with a slightly different flavor; highly recommended)

tamari soy sauce

umeboshi (salt-pickled plum)

For sweet flavor

See previous section: Natural Sweeteners

For sour flavor

brown rice vinegar
other naturally fermented vinegars
lemon

Herbs and Spices

The milder the better. Fiery hot and other extreme spices can cause an unbalanced condition. Fresh is best, but naturally dried herbs and spices are okay too. Use very small amounts.

basil

ginger (very good, especially fresh)

cinnamon

dill

garlic (if mild)

oregano

curry (if mild)

marjoram

thyme

bay leaves

tarragon

poppy seed

caraway seed

coriander seed

dry mustard

carob (for occasional use only, as a chocolate substitute)

Table Condiments

Choose your table condiments to add flavor to your
food and to increase its nutritional value. If using a
prepared condiment, such as pickles, mustard, or
mayonnaise, make sure it contains only the highest-
quality natural ingredients (natural sweeteners,
whole grain vinegar, and pure vegetable oils).

naturally fermented pickles and pickle relish

natural mustard

mayonnaise (eggless)

natural salad dressings

horseradish

sea salt

gomasio (roasted ground sesame seeds and sea salt:
nutty flavor, very good on cooked whole
grains)

furikake (roasted nori flakes, sesame seeds, and
miso)

powdered dulse

daikon pickles (daikon radish fermented in soy
sauce)

sauerkraut (salt-fermented cabbage)

umeboshi plums and umeboshi plum paste (Japanese pickled plum; tastes good with some whole grains and vegetables; also acts as a blood purifier. A single teaspoon can quickly heal certain ailments, such as muscle cramps and upset stomach.)

shiso leaf (beefsteak leaves fermented with umeboshi)

dried shiso leaf powder

tamari soy sauce (very salty; use sparingly at the table)

black pepper/white pepper (for occasional use; can be ground fresh at the table)

Beverages

It will help if you balance your intake of beverages the same way you would balance your intake of foods. How? By avoiding extremes.

The single best beverage is *water*. But make sure to drink only pure water from a well or spring, or filtered from the tap. Here are some other suggestions:

grain coffee

chicory root coffee

kukicha (roasted bancha twig tea)

non-caffeinated teas (roasted barley tea, mu tea, roasted brown rice tea, dandelion tea; for occasional use: mint tea, chamomile tea, wild berry teas)

club soda/seltzer water (chemical-free only)

mineral water (sparkling or nonsparkling)

homemade vegetable juices (occasionally)

soy milk (occasionally)

almond milk (occasionally)
fruit juices from locally grown fruit (occasionally, in small quantities)

Foods to Avoid

You should avoid the following foods because they cause too extreme or too unbalanced a condition. Eat these foods only one or two times a year or not at all.

Animal foods

red meat (beef, lamb, veal, pork)
certain seafoods (bluefish, crab, herring, lobster, sardines, swordfish, roe, red snapper, any smoked fish, caviar)

Vegetables

These are too high in acids or too expansive.
artichokes
asparagus
beets
chard
okra
rhubarb
spinach
zucchini

Spices

cayenne
saffron

nutmeg
cumin
cocoa (chocolate)

Fruits and nuts
Any that are not grown locally. See previous lists.

Oils and fats
cottonseed oil
palm/palm kernel oil
coconut oil
margarine
any processed oil, including all hydrogenated oils
animal shortenings (lard, bacon fat)

Condiments
most commercial mayonnaise
most commercial salad dressings
refined salt
commercial vinegars
brewer's yeast
catsup

Sweets and sugar foods (read labels)
jams and jellies
doughnuts, cakes, pies, pastries
chewing gum
ice cream
most breakfast cereals

most processed food (in cans and jars)

most commercially prepared dry foods ("instant" foods, mixes, other boxed foods)

most breads

many frozen foods

sugar (names of sugars to avoid in any product: granulated white sugar, powdered white sugar, brown sugar, turbinado sugar, raw sugar, sucrose, dextrose, maltose, fructose, lactose, glucose, corn syrup, corn sweetener)

honey (however, natural raw honey is a better choice than any refined sugar, above)

Beverages

alcoholic beverages

soft drinks and sodas

coffee

commercial teas

caffeinated teas

any extremely aromatic herbal teas

Refined and partial foods

any white flour product (white bread, white flour/semolina noodles and pastas, white flour pretzels and crackers, white flour pastries)

white rice

sugar (see "sweets and sugar foods")

vitamin and mineral supplements (except for special short-term needs described later in this chapter)

Chemicalized foods

any chemical additive (read labels)

dyed and colored foods (unfortunately, you will not find these listed on product labels; it's not required by law)

artificial sweeteners (any artificial sweetener: saccharine, sorbitol, aspartame, nutra-sweet. These deceive the body. From a taste-signal, the body prepares to deal with real sugar. Then, in the process of digestion, the body discovers it's dealing with a different chemical. The liver and kidneys are hardest hit, as they work overtime detoxifying this chemical from the blood.

Herbicides and pesticides (When buying fresh fruit and vegetables, buy "organic" and "organically grown" whenever possible. That way, you steer clear of foods that have been chemically treated in the growing process. These chemicals get into, and under, the skin of fresh foods and cannot be washed off completely. Also, when buying squash, cucumbers, rutabagas, and other root vegetables, avoid those that have been waxed. Finally, don't buy "fresh" fruits and vegetables that have been irradiated.)

Drugs and medications

any over-the-counter medication (Aspirin, cold and flu remedies, antacids, laxatives, decongestants treat symptoms only, not causes. Food is the best medicine. If you want to treat the underlying causes of your symptoms, change your diet.)

prescribed medications (These also treat only the symptoms, but much more serious symptoms. After quitting drinking, you need to get off any painkillers or mood-altering medication as soon as possible. But don't stop taking prescribed medication without a doctor's order, or without being under a specialist's care. To find other options, consult other specialists: MDs, dieticians, holistic healers, and so on. With a dietary plan such as the one in this book, and a specialist who knows your situation, you should be able to make a smooth transition.)

any illegal drugs (Any of the illegal drugs, including marijuana, creates too extreme a condition. They cause you to crave all kinds of extreme foods and become impossible to balance with a wholesome diet.)

HEALTHFUL WAYS OF COOKING AND EATING

How you eat is almost as important as what you eat. How you prepare your food and how you approach your food can make a world of difference. Here are some suggestions.

Use Various Methods of Preparation

You can gain additional variety in your meals and create different tastes for your foods by using various methods of preparation.

You can prepare a single food many different ways. With rice, for instance, you can *pressure cook* it or *boil* it and you will notice taste differences between the two. Once cooked, it can be added to *soup*, *stew*, or *salad* . . . or to bread dough or muffins for *baking* . . . pancake batter for *pan-frying* . . . or you could make a *stir-fry* with vegetables . . . or simply reheat the rice by *steaming.*

Here's a list to give you ideas:

Use regularly

pressure cooking (best with whole grains, some bean dishes)

boiling (with lid for grains and beans, without lid for vegetables)

pan-frying/sautéing (with a small amount of oil, no water; good for fish, pancakes, and vegetables, especially onion or other root vegetables or summer squash)

stir-frying (brown ingredients, add small amount of water, then simmer covered for a few minutes; good for vegetables, fried grains, or grain with vegetable dishes.)

steaming (good for vegetables, especially dark green leafy vegetables, winter squash, bush or pole beans)

baking (good for squash, fish, vegetable casseroles, chicken)

stews (the works: vegetables, grains, and beans, even whole grain noodles, and thickened with kuzu or arrowroot)

salads (combinations of raw and cooked)

soups (made mainly with vegetables, often with the addition of whole grains or beans; best if flavored with miso or tamari soy sauce)

Use only occasionally

broiling (fish)

deep-frying (chicken or tempura vegetables)

Use the Best Cookware

When you use top-quality cookware, your meals will taste better and be healthier too. As soon as possible, throw away any poor-quality cookware and go buy whatever you need.

What's best? Stainless steel and cast iron cookware. Also very good: enamel-coated cast iron, enamel-coated stainless steel, earthenware, and Pyrex.

Avoid aluminum, any nonstick cookware, and copper. Every time you cook with these implements, some molecules from them get into the food, making your food taste slightly metallic or "tinny" and putting stress on your body. These substances can reach toxic levels quickly. In the case of aluminum, the body has trouble eliminating this metal. It builds in the tissue and may cause long-term problems. For instance, aluminum has been linked to Alzheimer's disease. Research shows that the brain tissue of those who died of Alzheimer's has, on the average, four times the amount of aluminum as a normal brain.

When you use cast iron cookware, some of the iron gets into your food also. Major difference: The iron is good for you.

For the same reasons, don't store food in metal or plastic containers. Metal and plastic compounds can leach into your foods. Tests show the polyvinyl chlorides (PVCs) in plastics can be dangerous to your health. For storing food, use nonleaded ceramic, wood, or glass.

Chew Well

Many Americans not only eat fast food, they eat food fast. Often we gulp our meals, hardly even tasting the food.

Unfortunately, this taxes our systems, resulting in poor or incomplete digestion and malabsorption of nutrients. The reason? Digestion begins in the mouth. Saliva mixes with food to start the long process of digestion. It's the first key ingredient in the breakdown of food. In addition, the more we break down the food with our teeth, the more complete our total digestion will be. When we chew well, food remains in the mouth longer and more saliva is produced. That means the body can absorb and use more nutrients for each mouthful.

You can improve digestion 100% if you begin to chew your food well. Some authorities recommend you chew every mouthful 100 to 200 times. I recommend you start with 25 to 50.

Or try this: Chew as much as necessary to thoroughly pulverize your food. The more liquid your food is when you swallow it, the better.

Gandhi said, "You must chew your drinks and drink your foods." You'll find every meal more satisfying when you do.

Eat Only When Hungry

Some people feel a craving to eat all the time, especially after quitting an addiction such as drinking or smoking. You tend to fill the gap with food.

How do you break the habit? Best way: Retrain your body. Listen to your inner needs; listen to your body's true signals for hunger. And learn to pay attention.

Sometimes it is a good idea to wait five or six hours between meals, or to fast for a whole day. This can help you focus attention on your inner sensations of hunger.

Don't eat just because "it's time to eat," but only

when you're hungry. You will soon learn to distinguish true hunger from "addictive hunger."

When You Are Hungry, Eat

When you feel hungry, truly hungry, you should eat. And don't wait too long.

Why this rule? It's because your hypoglycemia may cause nervousness if you wait too long between meals. You can get fidgety, even have the shakes. You may get angry at yourself and people around you. You can experience headache, tension, the whole list of hypoglycemic symptoms.

If you feel hungry, eat. Sometimes a small healthy snack will do. If you're really hungry, eat a regular meal.

To control hypoglycemia, many health practitioners recommend eating six meals a day. How? Just plan your day to include six small meals. In practice, you can plan for three regular meals, three healthy snacks, and no sugar foods. With a plan like this, your blood sugar will remain at a more constant level all day long. That means your emotions will remain fairly steady as well.

The six-meal-a-day plan works very well. Especially when you first quit drinking—while your body is adjusting to a new diet—plan to eat many small meals each day. It will help you over the hump. It will help you make your initial adjustment to a life without drinking.

Relax When You Eat

Sounds simple, right? It may not be. Many of us spent our first 18 or so years in families where a great amount of tension surrounded every meal. Now, whenever we begin to eat, even when we're alone, we feel uptight.

If you relax when you eat, your digestion will be much more efficient. You will tend not to eat too much. And you will enjoy your food much more.

How can you learn this? First, simply be aware while you eat. Eat slowly. Allow yourself to enter a calm and peaceful state. Second, use some special techniques. Any of the relaxation techniques discussed in Chapter 7 can help immensely.

Don't Eat Two to Three Hours Before Bedtime

Here's a simple rule that can help you sleep better and help you feel better the next day. Don't eat before bedtime. And don't get up to eat in the middle of the night.

The reason? In sleep, your bodily functions slow down. You digest food more slowly. So if you eat soon before sleep, the food remains undigested for a longer period of time. How does this affect you? Since digestion competes with sleep, your sleep becomes more restless. What's worse, you may still feel full in the morning and fatigued before the day begins.

When you first begin to change, you will probably find it difficult to avoid food for two to three hours before bedtime. But stay with it. It's a habit you can change, and a peaceful night's sleep can be well worth the effort.

When You Eat, Do Not Overeat

Perhaps as important as what you eat is how much. When you eat too much, you strain all the digestive organs, especially the liver.

When you overeat, you tend to feel sluggish, tired, or sleepy. You may also feel irritable, or tend to anger quickly.

Nonetheless, overeating may be hard to cure. Why? When you quit drinking, overeating comes naturally. You may start eating excess food at meals and excess food between meals. What to do? Here's a helpful way to approach it:

Take your time. At every meal or snack, take your time. Relax. Chew well. As you eat, listen to your body. Listen closely. Your body will signal when it's had enough.

Practice eating less. What happens if you don't hear the signal or if, when you hear the signal, you've already eaten too much? In this case, practice eating a certain amount, a normal meal with small to average servings. When you've finished this, stop. Don't go for seconds. Get up from the table and begin doing something else. After a few minutes, you will forget about eating. Now, how do you feel? Lighter? More peaceful? Stronger?

How much should you eat at any meal? It's up to you. Take time to learn your body's inner needs and what's best for you. On this subject, here's an old proverb from the Talmud that may help: "In eating, a third of the stomach should be filled with food, a third with drink, and the rest left empty."

TO SUPPLEMENT OR NOT TO SUPPLEMENT

For 50,000 years of human history, we have gotten our essential nutrients from the food we eat. But now we have another option. Essential nutrients are available in the form of supplements.

What are supplements? Supplements, in pills or powders, offer concentrated forms of vitamins, minerals, proteins (amino acids), and other essential bodybuilders.

Where do supplements come from? Food. Like white sugar and white flour, supplements are highly refined food products. Manufacturers start with a whole food and chemically or mechanically remove everything except the desired product.

The best source of nutrients is still food. When you eat whole (unrefined) foods, you get the important vitamins, minerals, and proteins, plus the fiber, the carbohydrates, the essential oils, and the all-important enzymes to help your body digest and absorb the nutrients.

But what if your body has been abused by years and years of unbalanced diet, heavy drinking, and malabsorption of nutrients? Certainly you will need some time to adapt to health. It may take a few weeks before your body can begin absorbing essential nutrients from the food you eat.

So as soon as you quit drinking, you might try certain supplements to restore your vitamin and mineral levels. Like jump-starting a car, it can give your body a quick boost and get you back on the right road.

Once you reestablish your ability to absorb nutrients, you should stop using supplements. This may take only a few weeks. Then your body can begin doing the work it was designed to do: gaining its nutrients from food.

Guidelines for Supplements

Vitamin C.   Helps with liver detox. Some treatment specialists recommend 4,000 to 5,000 mg a day. But too much can cause its own toxic reaction. I recommend 500 to 1000 mg a day for the first two weeks. Then quit it, or take only 50 to 100 mg a day as a supplement. The RDA (recommended daily allowance) for vitamin C is 60 mg. For comparison, one medium stalk of cooked broccoli has 160 mg of vitamin C, one cup of cooked cauliflower flowerets has 69 mg, one cup of cooked kale, collards, or turnip greens has 100 mg, and one cup of chopped raw parsley has 100 mg.

Silymarin. Also helps with liver detox. This extract of milk thistle has been shown to improve the liver's efficiency. You may try it as a supplement before meals for the first two weeks. Then stop taking it, or reduce intake to one meal a day or one meal every other day.

Glutamine. Recommended by many researchers, this amino acid can curb the craving for alcohol, drugs, and sugar. If you want to try it, take 500 mg two or three times a day between meals.

Like vitamins and minerals, however, amino acids work together. If you artificially raise one, others will be depleted. That means that while taking glutamine, you may find yourself craving various protein foods that contain glutamine in relatively low proportions compared to other amino acids.

Yet glutamine has a proven value. Some studies show it can curb cravings for alcohol after you quit drinking. Other studies show it can curb the craving to drink even before you quit drinking.

But all studies show it works *only for some drinkers*. For this reason, if you decide to try it, try it for a day or two first, to see whether it works for you.

Better yet, get it from natural sources. These include whole wheat, carrots, radishes, and cabbage.

Dosages. Excessive alcohol consumption depletes vitamins (especially B vitamins) and minerals. Yet supplementing these can be tricky. Why? You can overdose on supplements. Too much of certain supplements can cause a toxic reaction. For this reason, you need to take low doses (or no doses) of vitamins A, D, and E. Secondly, vitamins and minerals work together. Too much of one will deplete the body's supply of another.

Some manufacturers have balanced the vitamins and minerals in their multivitamin tablets to match the proportions of vitamins and minerals found in the body. These supplements are the best. Buy them in health food stores, not grocery stores or pharmacies. The health-food-store product will come in a base free of sugar, salt, starch, artificial ingredients, and additives.

For comparison, here's a list of all the ingredients you want, and approximate amounts of each:

vitamin A	5,000	IU (international units)
vitamin D	100	IU
vitamin E	100	IU
vitamin C	500	mg
vitamin B-1	50	mg
vitamin B-2	50	mg
vitamin B-3	100	mg
vitamin B-6	50	mg
vitamin B-12	50	mcg (micrograms)

folic acid	0.4	mg
pantothenic acid	100	mg
biotin	100	mcg
choline	100	mg
inositol	100	mg
vitamin K	10	mcg
bioflavinoids (rutin, hesperidin)	100	mcg
calcium	100	mg
chromium	50	mcg
copper	2	mg
iodine	150	mcg
iron	18	mg
magnesium	100	mg
manganese	5	mg
potassium	100	mg
selenium	50	mcg
zinc	20	mg

You may try a vitamin/mineral supplement, such as the one listed above, for the first few weeks after you quit drinking. This will replenish depleted supplies and help your body relearn the absorption of vitamins and minerals. Then stop taking it and get all your appropriate nutrients from good food.

Now How Do You Answer?

To supplement or not to supplement? If you take my advice, you'll supplement for two or three weeks, maybe a month, while in transition from heavy drinking to a whole-foods diet. Two exceptions: If you can't make the change to a whole-foods diet (and especially if you eat a lot of junk food), I recommend you keep taking supplements. Second, I recommend you start taking supplements before you quit drinking and continue taking them until you make the diet change. The alcoholic diet is about the worst there is and needs as much help as it can get.

If you don't like my advice, you can choose any of these other options:

Long-term supplementation. Some researchers and treatment specialists recommend the long-term use of supplements. For three approaches see:

> *Alcoholism, The Biochemical Connection: A Breakthrough Seven-Week Self-Treatment Program* by Joan Mathews-Larsen, Ph.D. New York: Villard Books, 1992.

> *The Hidden Addiction, and How to Get Free* by Janice Phelps, MD, and Alan Nourse, MD. Boston: Little, Brown, 1986.

> *Eating Right to Live Sober* by Katherine Ketcham and L. Ann Mueller, MD. New York: New American Library, 1983.

Optional short-term supplementation. Some authorities recommend this approach, which is similar to mine. See two variations in the following:

> *Staying Sober: A Nutrition and Exercise Program for the Recovering Alcoholic* by Judy Myers with Maribeth Mellin. New York: Congdon & Weed, 1987.

Good Food for a Sober Life by Jack Mumey and
    Anne Hatcher, Ed.D., RD. Chicago: Contem-
    porary Books, 1987.

No supplements. Other specialists recommend no
supplements whatsoever. See, for instance:

Food and Healing by Annemarie Colbin. New
    York: Ballantine Books, 1986.
Healing Ourselves by Naboru Muramoto with
    Michel Abehsera. New York: Avon Books,
    1973.

HOW TO MAKE THE CHANGE

Get Into Cooking

You will need to take some extra time with cooking.
This may be a burden at first. But with a little patience and perhaps a slightly different perspective,
you can learn to enjoy it.

Remember to plan ahead. A bean dish from
scratch (starting with dried beans) takes about two
hours to cook. Whole grains usually take one hour.
But here's the good news: You don't have to watch
these dishes cook. Just check on them every half-hour
or so. Also, if you make a big potful, it saves time. The
next few days, you can reheat leftovers in minutes for
many different dishes.

When you plan ahead, everything seems to take
less time. At least you know what to expect and can
accept it.

Overall, you probably will be spending more time
preparing meals. You may even resent having to
spend the extra time. I know I did. Yet here's the

thought that helped me: For every hour I spent preparing healthy meals, I kept telling myself I would gain three extra hours on the total length of my life. And I reminded myself that my life would be a healthier life as well.

Try Various Recipes

Starting a new diet can be viewed as a great adventure. So many new foods! So many new ways to prepare them!

It's your opportunity to try as many new recipes as you can. For the first few months, try five to ten new recipes or cooking styles each week. You'll enjoy the variety and become quickly proficient in the new diet.

Here are some recommended cookbooks using whole foods and natural, healthy ingredients:

The Self-Healing Cookbook by Kristina Turner. Vashon Island, WA: Earthtones Press, 1989 (good starter book).

Macrobiotic Cooking for Everyone by Edward and Wendy Esko. Tokyo: Japan Publications, 1980. (good starter book).

Introducing Macrobiotic Cooking by Wendy Esko. Tokyo: Japan Publications, 1983 (good starter book).

The Book of Whole Meals: A Seasonal Guide to Assembling Balanced Vegetarian Breakfasts, Lunches, and Dinners by Annemarie Colbin. New York: Ballantine Books, 1983.

Whole World Cookbook: International Macrobiotic Cuisine by the editors of *East West Journal*. Wayne, NJ: Avery Publishing Group, 1984.

Deliciously Simple: Quick and Easy, Low-Sodium, Low-Fat, Low-Cholesterol, Low-Sugar Meals by Harriet Roth (former director of Pritikin Longevity Center). New York: New American Library, 1986.

How to Cook with Miso by Aveline Kushi. Tokyo: Japan Publications, 1978.

The Do of Cooking by Cornelia Aihara. Oroville, CA: GOMF Press, 1982 (very advanced).

The Vegetarian Epicure (two volumes) by Anna Thomas. New York: Knopf, 1978.

Still Life with Menu by Mollie Katzen. Berkeley, CA: Ten Speed Press, 1988. (Or try *The Enchanted Broccoli Forest* or *The Moosewood Cookbook*, also by Mollie Katzen.)

The Gradual Vegetarian by Lisa Tracy. New York: Dell, 1985. (This book gives a great three-step method for making a gradual change from a meat-based diet.)

Get Acquainted with New Foods

How do you get acquainted with new foods? Learn where to shop and what to look for.

Where to shop. Some supermarkets now carry whole grains, dried beans, organically grown produce, and other "health food" items. Look for these sections in your supermarket.

And, in most areas, you can find health food stores and natural-food cooperatives. Check them out. Many great selections are available at these stores, plus the workers there can be very helpful. Begin shopping at these alternative food stores for a good portion of your supplies.

Of course, if you live near any organic farmers, you may want to buy some of the foods they grow and sell at roadside stands. Or else grow your own. If you start your own garden, you can enjoy high-quality foods and get some exercise too. A great combination!

What to look for. When you shop, read labels. Look for the very best ingredients: no chemical additives, no preservatives, no refined foods (such as sugar and white flour), and no artificial ingredients. Pay top dollar to get the best quality. Don't skimp on the food you eat. After all, the food you select will enrich your very life.

What If You Don't Like the New Foods?

At first you may not like many of the new foods. Whenever making a major dietary change, most people have the same problem. But after a while, you will adjust to new tastes and respond to new feelings aroused by foods.

We must acquire a taste for some things. For instance, most of us didn't like alcohol the first time we tried it. But because we thought it was cool or made us look more adult, we kept drinking until we learned to like it.

With the new diet, keep reminding yourself that these foods will help you look younger, regain your health, and feel better. These reminders, in turn, will spark your desire to stay with the new foods.

Moreover, it doesn't take too long before you begin to taste the wholesome goodness of these foods. Give your taste buds a little time to adjust. Soon you will find many favorite foods on the new menu, foods you will like as much as, if not more than, your current favorite foods.

But you may absolutely dislike certain aspects of this diet. If so, don't worry. You can choose another special diet.

One caution, however: Choose a diet for health. Do not choose a diet for weight reduction. Why? Weight-loss diets tend to be extremely unbalanced in one way or another. In the long run, these diets can cause serious problems. Anyway, on a healthy diet, your body finds its own best weight, whatever is fit and trim for you.

Here are some healthy diet alternatives:

- The Pritikin Diet. See *The Pritikin Program for Diet and Exercise* by Nathan Pritikin with Patrick McGrady, Jr. New York: Grosset & Dunlap, 1979.
- Raw foods diet to cure hypoglycemia. See *Hypoglycemia: A Better Approach* by Dr. Paavo Airola. Phoenix, AZ: Health Plus Publishers, 1977.
- Vegetarian. See *Transition to Vegetarianism* by Rudolph Ballentine, MD. Honesdale, PA: Himalayan International Institute, 1987.

Or try one of these new books on dietary cure for alcoholics:

The Hidden Addiction and How to Get Free by Janice Phelps, MD, and Alan Nourse, MD. Boston: Little, Brown, 1986.

Good Food for a Sober Life by Jack Mumey and Anne Hatcher, Ed.D., RD. Chicago: Contemporary Books, 1987.

Eating Right to Live Sober by Katherine Ketcham and L. Ann Mueller, MD. New York: New American Library, 1983.

Need More Support?

Changing your diet takes a great deal of inner strength. Some people go it alone without any problem, while others do better with outside support.

If you need support, here are four places to look:

Start at home. Get your spouse, your family, or your roommates on your side. Explain that you're going to start eating healthy foods. Invite them to do the same. Tell them that they too can gain greater strength, have more energy, and live longer, healthier lives if they will join you.

Even then, you may not get too many takers. Just like you, they have become addicted to the foods they eat. And most people don't want to give up those foods, no matter how much you try to convince them of the damage they cause.

So be prepared. You may have to go it alone at home. Plan to make separate meals from your spouse, your family, or roommates, if they don't want to participate. But watch how they continue to be very curious about what you eat and watch how you gradually win them over in the long run.

Try a support group. In most areas you will find various "natural foods" groups, such as Pritikin groups, vegetarian groups, and macrobiotic groups. These groups meet regularly, usually to share a meal and exchange good thoughts.

Try cooking classes. Similar to joining a support group, except you will meet in a kitchen. Here you can gain helpful hints on cooking and learn to make many interesting recipes.

Go to a dietary counselor. A dietary counselor will give you individual attention and a personalized diet to meet your specific needs. When you go, be sure to provide accurate information. For instance: how long you have been a heavy drinker, what kind of health ailments you have, what kind of foods you eat, and so on.

When selecting a nutritionist, make sure he or she steers away from any refined or processed foods. Also, make sure this nutritionist doesn't advocate the "Four Food Groups" classification system. Too many inconsistencies arise from this system. Of course, it has now been officially replaced by the "Food Pyramid." The pyramid is a better system. It can bring you into better health than the Four Food Groups—but only slightly better. The reason? The pyramid offers better guidelines for selecting foods, but it doesn't go far enough in eliminating the poor-quality foods. Actually, you can gain greater health from other types of diet.

Here are some suggested types of dietary counselors:

> holistic health practitioners
>
> macrobiotic dietary counselors (at East-West Centers across the nation)
>
> "whole foods" nutritionists
>
> Pritikin health counselors

What About Dining Out?

When on a health-food diet in a junk-food world, dining out can be a nightmare.

The good news: You can now find more and more vegetarian and natural-foods restaurants. Go to these as much as possible. Take a little extra time out of your schedule if necessary.

The bad news: It's not always possible to get to a good restaurant.

Solution: Get a salad. Even fast food restaurants offer salads. Other possibilities: side dishes of vegetables (any cooked vegetables or cole slaw, but not french fries), fish, chicken salad, or chicken (not deep-fat fried).

How to Begin a New Diet

Change gradually or all at once? Which kind of person are you? Some people like to ease into things. Others prefer to make sweeping changes without looking back. When quitting coffee, for instance, some folks gradually decrease their consumption little by little over a period of months. Others simply can't decrease their consumption slowly. It's all-or-nothing for them. Even if they drink five to ten cups a day, they need to quit it all at once—cold turkey.

What will be easiest for you?

Make a decision now concerning how to start your new diet. Gradually? Or all at once?

When to make the change. You can change some parts of your diet before you quit drinking, and change other parts later. If you want to make some changes before you quit drinking, here are the easiest things to do first:

- Stop eating white flour products and white rice; start eating whole wheat products and whole rice.
- Stop eating chemicalized foods: artificial flavors, artificial sugars, chemical additives, preservatives.
- Stop sweets and sugar foods. (You won't be able

to do this cleanly, because alcohol converts to
sugar in the body. If it's a choice between having
something sweet or drinking alcohol, choose the
sweet.)

- Cut out nicotine.
- Cut out caffeine. (Don't substitute decaffeinated
  coffees or teas. These products still contain
  some caffeine. What's worse, they are loaded
  with chemicals from the manufacturing process, with one exception: organically grown coffee, decaffeinated with the patented "Swiss
  water process.")
- Add as many vegetables to your menu as you
  can, especially dark green leafy vegetables.

Note: You will not be able to change all of your
diet *before* you quit drinking. The reason? Alcohol
keeps your diet too unbalanced. Alcohol is so extremely expansive, you will need strong contractive
foods to balance it; for instance, meats, eggs, salty
foods.

But by changing some things before you quit
drinking, you can get a head start on the new diet.
This will help, especially if you are someone who
likes to change gradually. Even if you prefer to change
things all at once, you can view each category separately. For instance, you can change from white flour
products to no white flour products . . . you can quit
coffee or cigarettes completely . . . or quit chemicals
all at once . . . and so on.

Nevertheless, if you prefer to wait until you quit
drinking and do *everything* at once, do that. But remember, do not try to quit drinking gradually. Quit it
completely and change completely to your new diet at
that time.

HOW TO HANDLE CRAVINGS

What are cravings? What can you do about them? And can you ever cheat by having some of the food (or drug) you're craving?

What Are Cravings?

Cravings stir you. They nag you and try to cloud your mind. Cravings frighten you and fight with you, attempting to control your behavior.

When you quit drinking you will experience cravings for alcohol. When you quit sweets, you will crave sweets. Quit meats and you will crave them. When you quit anything your body has adjusted to, you'll get cravings for it.

In the body, cravings are biochemical expectations. Each of us craves different things because each body has a certain biochemistry which is different from everyone else's. In part, you create your own internal biochemistry, as it depends on the kinds of foods you eat and on the kinds of drugs you take. Yet all human bodies are the same in some ways. For instance, our bodies expect to get a certain set of biochemical nutrients from our diets. Take something away and the body will notice immediately. It will "think" it's missing something. This feeling inside, of something missing, is what we call craving.

Cravings can be of two kinds. You can crave things your body needs (vitamins, minerals, proteins, oils, and carbohydrates from various sources). Or you can crave things you don't need (alcohol, drugs, sweets and sugar foods).

Both kinds of cravings depend on the body's biochemical expectations. For instance, alcohol and drugs raise endorphins in the brain, biochemically causing calmness, pleasure, and euphoria. The body craves the alcohol or the drug on the expectation that pleasurable sensations will follow each time. Now let's take a look at the other kind of craving. Let's say you drink orange juice frequently and orange juice in your diet has become a primary source of vitamin C. This means that whenever your body needs vitamin C, you will begin craving orange juice. If your body had been accustomed to getting vitamin C from broccoli and dark green leafy vegetables, whenever your body got low on vitamin C, you would begin craving these particular vegetables.

Now for a moment imagine what it would take for you to change. Could you teach your body not to crave the orange juice when needing vitamin C and to crave the broccoli and dark green leaves instead? Try it. You'll notice it takes a long time for the body to learn this replacement.

That's why staying on a new diet can be so difficult. The body keeps craving foods from the old diet. This craving will persist until your body adjusts to gaining its essential nutrients from the new foods.

A suggestion: When you quit drinking, change to your new diet the same day. That way your cravings for food and alcohol get mixed. What's so good about this? Since food cravings tend to overcome alcohol cravings, you won't notice your alcohol cravings as much. And this makes quitting so much easier.

What to Do About Cravings?

For food cravings: Stay with the new diet and wait them out. Give yourself some time. Often the body makes an adjustment on its own.

While waiting, try this: When experiencing a food

craving, consider what your body is telling you. Feel it. What does the body want? What food in the new diet might satisfy the craving? When you do this you will discover more about the inner workings of your body. And you'll learn what kind of foods are good for you.

For alcohol cravings: Use any way you can to reduce your cravings for alcohol. Use the dietary techniques you learned in this chapter, and the exercise and relaxation techniques you'll learn in the next chapter.

Meanwhile, beware of other excesses. When you quit drinking, you will tend to fill in the gap with other drugs, and you may start overeating. You will tend to eat more sweets, smoke more cigarettes, drink more coffee, or take more over-the-counter medications, such as aspirin. Avoid this tendency as much as possible. It will just keep you craving alcohol for a longer period of time after you quit drinking.

Finally, here are the most important dietary changes to reduce cravings when you quit drinking: Reduce your intake of animal protein. The less meat and eggs you eat, the less you will crave alcohol. Increase your intake of whole grains, fruits, and vegetables.

In general, simply stay with the new diet as strictly as you can. Gradually your body will adjust to the new foods and your cravings will diminish. Immediately you will benefit from greater nutrition. As this happens, you'll gain more strength, stamina, and willpower.

When to Cheat?

Can you ever give in to your cravings without compromising your health? Yes . . . and no.

Yes, you can give in to food cravings under certain circumstances. No, you can't give in to alcohol or drug cravings.

Here are some guidelines: If cravings persist, wait at least two full days for food cravings and four full days for sweets cravings. Then if you're still craving, allow yourself to have some. And enjoy it . . . like giving yourself a treat. But study it too. Whether it's a steak or ice cream, you may notice, over time, you begin liking these treats less and less.

Special stop-gap measure when craving alcohol: Don't give in to an alcohol craving. Wait . . . do exercises . . . put it off another day . . . do more exercises and wait some more. But if you're having an outrageous craving for alcohol, to the point where you can't control it, *have something sweet.*

Only problem: In a couple of hours you will probably get the craving again. So don't use this method too often; otherwise, you reduce its effectiveness. Remember, the sweets addiction is a result of alcohol addiction. You need to quit sweets in order to improve your health and strengthen your nervous system. So cheat with sweets only under dire circumstances. If it's a matter of having a drink or having a quart of ice cream, have the ice cream.

Practice #4

Start Your New Diet

Instructions: If you've already quit drinking, start your new diet now. Get into it as quickly as you can, but as gradually as you need to.

If you haven't quit drinking, you can start making some of the recommended changes. Even if you don't make the dietary changes immediately, take time to get the cookbooks, get acquainted with new foods and food stores . . . and begin planning. Plan to stop drinking soon and start eating for health at the same time.

CHAPTER 7

Building Inner Strength

Consciousness of our powers increases them.
—*Vauvenargues*

W hat's the single most important thing you can do after you quit drinking? Return to health as quickly as possible. Why? Health means strength. By returning to health, you gain both physical and mental strength. And both kinds of strength will help you abstain from drinking.

As you become stronger, you become more aware, more sensitive. You gain the power to make more decisions. You actually gain consciousness. It's like a new awakening. Building your inner strength helps you build a powerful awareness of your true inner self.

How do you build your strength? The same way you build your health: through diet and exercise. With proper diet and sufficient exercise, you become strong and healthy.

Yet anyone who has been an excessive drinker has

much to overcome. Why? Because alcohol takes something from you. Instead of building inner strength, it tears your insides apart and deadens your consciousness. You may feel powerful when you're high, but it's a false power. When you come down, you feel nervous, depressed, and lost.

For those addicted to alcohol, poor health is like a cloud surrounding you—a cloud that gets darker and darker. When you quit your addiction, the cloud slowly clears. As you regain health, you begin to see again. Everything appears fresh and new. There is probably no better feeling in the world than the feeling of regaining your health.

To be sure, good health acts as its own reward. Health brings happiness. The healthier you become, the happier you will feel—and the less you will want to drink.

So energize yourself. Renew yourself. Regain your health as soon as possible.

We've looked at dietary ways to improve your health. Now let's look at exercise. You can work with two kinds of exercise: physical and mental. Physical exercise strengthens your heart, improves your circulation, and gives you more energy. Mental exercise— changing your way of thinking—helps you manage stress, feel relaxed, and become more self-confident.

In this chapter, you will discover how to:

- energize yourself with exercise.
- calm yourself with relaxation techniques.
- improve your self-image with assertiveness skills.
- reduce inner tension with stress management and coping techniques.
- renew human caring through friendship.

EXERCISE

Action is the proper fruit of knowledge.
　　　　　　　　　　　—*Thomas Fuller, MD*

Physical exercise builds physical strength. With exercise, your muscles improve, your body tone improves, even your internal organs get stronger.

But here's something you may not know: Physical exercise builds mental strength as well. It's true. Scientists have pinpointed a biochemical reason for this. Vigorous physical activity causes the body to produce endorphins, the body's natural tranquilizers, which act on brain cells and nerve cells. They calm you as powerfully as related chemicals: morphine and the isoquinolines. (Isoquinolines, remember, cause the sedative effect during excessive alcohol consumption.)

So to find peace and calm when you quit drinking, get into exercise. It has a naturally tranquilizing effect. Without physical exercise, you can become nervous and depressed, or your life may seem dreary and dull. Endorphins, however, create a natural high. These powerful biochemicals can help you beat depression and stave off anxiety.

Tennyson once said, "I myself must mix with action, lest I wither by despair." This holds true for everyone. So when you quit drinking, use the extra time you gain to become as active as you can.

How do you get active? Plan your own exercise program, one that will work for you. Then begin doing it.

Worksheet #6

Plan Your Own Exercise Program

Physical exercise not only helps build health and inner
strength, it's one of the most powerful tools to help beat
depression. With this worksheet, you will plan for two
kinds of physical exercise: aerobic exercise and casual exercise. Make sure to add both to your personal program for
quitting drinking.

Aerobic Exercise

Aerobic exercise is highly active. It's a fast physical workout that lasts 20 to 30 minutes without interruption. This
kind of exercise strengthens your heart and circulation and
leaves you feeling relaxed for 12 to 24 hours.

Aerobic exercise gives you the greatest production of
endorphins, the body's natural tranquilizers. Perhaps
you've heard of "runner's high." This is the point in your
workout when you begin to feel euphoric, usually after 20
to 30 minutes of vigorous activity.

You will gain the greatest benefits by planning three
or four aerobic workouts a week. Scientific studies show
that the heart begins to lose the benefits of conditioning
when more than two days go by without exercise. So if
you exercise on Monday, you will need to exercise again
by Wednesday and no later than Thursday. That way, you
stay in shape and keep your heart fit.

When selecting exercises, be sure to choose those that
match your way of life, that are fun for you and easy to do.
And keep in mind that you don't have to do the same
thing all the time. You have many options. For instance,
let's say you already play soccer on Saturdays; then maybe
you can plan a brisk walk for Mondays, go jogging on Tues-
days, and workout on the rowing machine in your basement on Thursdays.

By the way, it's a good idea to plan for four aerobic
workouts each week. That way, if you miss one, you still
achieve the minimum of three workouts. For instance, in
the preceding example, suppose it was raining cats and

dogs on Monday and you missed your walk. You still have your run planned for the next day, so you meet minimum requirements. But if it was pouring the next day too, you can't let this day go by—so start jogging in place or go down to the basement and workout on the rowing machine.

Use the following checklist to choose your exercises. Then use the weekly schedule to plan a typical week.

Checklist of Aerobic Activities

To qualify, all of the following must be done briskly for a minimum of 20 minutes without interruption.

Exercise:

- ☐ jogging/running
- ☐ running in place
- ☐ walking/hiking
- ☐ swimming
- ☐ rowing/rowing machine
- ☐ canoeing/kayaking
- ☐ bicycling/bicycle machine
- ☐ cross-country skiing/skiing machine
- ☐ trampoline
- ☐ dancing (vigorous)
- ☐ aerobic exercise classes
- ☐ roller skating
- ☐ ice skating
- ☐ indoor workout and conditioning machines
- ☐ jumping rope
- ☐ any vigorous exercise routine or workout

Some sports may qualify:

- ☐ ice hockey
- ☐ basketball (if you play a nonstop full-court game)
- ☐ soccer
- ☐ tennis (singles)
- ☐ handball/racquetball
- ☐ downhill skiing

Other possibilities:

- ☐ mowing lawn (No, riding mowers don't count)
- ☐ gardening (active phases such as hand-hoeing a row for planting, shoveling mulch)
- ☐ splitting wood
- ☐ shoveling snow
- ☐ painting a room
- ☐ trimming a hedge
- ☐ your choice: _____

Remember, the main test for aerobic exercise: You must stay continuously active in the exercise for at least 20 minutes.

Weekly Schedule

Select four days of the week when you can schedule 30 minutes for an aerobic workout. Then set the time you will do the workout. It can be a different time each day. Just make sure you choose times when you are free. Write the times exactly. For instance, Monday you may want to workout in the morning, 7–7:30 A.M.; Wednesday you may choose the late afternoon, 5–5:30 P.M. Now write in the exercise you will do at these times. The first exercise you write will be your preferred exercise for that time. Then write in a backup exercise. This will be the exercise you will do in case you can not do your preferred exercise.

	Time of Day	Exercise	Backup Exercise
Mon	_____	_____	_____
Tue	_____	_____	_____
Wed	_____	_____	_____
Thu	_____	_____	_____
Fri	_____	_____	_____
Sat	_____	_____	_____
Sun	_____	_____	_____

*One precaution about a 20 to 30-minute nonstop work-
out:* You will probably need to work your way up to a 20-
to 30-minute nonstop workout. Start slowly and build
your way up. If you have any soreness or pains, particularly chest pains, stop! Remember, it takes time to get in
shape. Find your own pace and don't push yourself.

If you have any serious physical problems, you may
need specific guidelines for exercise. Consult with your
doctor. If you are 35 years old or older, make sure to have a
medical checkup before you begin.

Give Yourself Time to Gain the Benefits

Although exercise brings about a natural high, it takes a
while before you can feel this benefit clearly. You need to
recondition your body, get your body into training. You'll
notice that the effects of exercise are cumulative. They get
stronger the longer you've been at it.

It takes a while to break old patterns. Alcohol brings
an instant high; if your body has become adjusted to alcohol, all your cells have become lazy. They get high without having to perform any activity. But this lethargy at the
cellular level, in the long run, causes disease.

Activity brings health. So give yourself time. The benefits—euphoria and relaxation—come gradually, but are
well worth it.

Also keep in mind that the high you get from exercise
may not feel as high as the high you get from alcohol. But
the exercise high is solid. You don't feel spaced out or out
of control. Plus the exercise high stays with you, and
there's no hangover.

One Myth

Many people feel that physical exercise wears you out.
This is a myth that needs to be dispelled. Physical exercise
actually gives you more energy throughout the day. The
more you do, the more you can do.

By the same token, the less you do, the less you can
do. If you lounge around, that's all your body will want to
do. You will feel more tired all the time. You will actually
need more sleep. You will feel sick more often, and actu-

ally get sick more often. You will also feel depressed, often seriously depressed, most of the time.

If you want to put it to a test, try this: Work out for three days and see how you feel. Then lie around for the same amount of time and compare your feelings.

You'll notice that physical exercise doesn't wear you out. Rather, it improves your health, vitality, and energy.

Gaining Momentum

It may take you a while to build momentum, to get yourself to the point where exercise feels natural. But rest assured, it will happen. You may have to force yourself at first, but after a while you will find yourself actually wanting to exercise.

Remember, the more you do, the more you can do. Your body adjusts. After a while your body gets into a rhythm and doesn't want to miss any of your workouts.

That's when you have momentum on your side. Once you get your exercise going on a fairly steady, regular basis, you tend to keep it going. So stay with your program long enough to get the momentum working for you. Then everything gets easier.

Casual Exercise

Any physical activity not vigorous enough or not long enough to be considered aerobic may be called a casual exercise. Our lives are filled with casual exercise. Just walking from room to room is a casual exercise.

The worst thing you can do is lie around. Why? You'll get depressed—and stay that way. It's a vicious circle: Lying around makes you depressed, and what's the only thing you want to do when you get depressed? Lie around.

So don't get caught in this trap. Plan to be as active as you can. Instead of using your car, walk or ride your bike. Instead of escalators or elevators, take the stairs. As much as possible, use your own human power instead of machines. Use hand saws instead of power saws, push mowers instead of riding mowers; wash the dishes by hand instead of using a dishwasher, and so on.

Also, plan to do stretching exercises, especially yoga.

Yoga is just about the best all-around exercise you can do. (For more details on yoga, see the next section, Relaxation Techniques.)

Checklist of Casual Exercises

- ☐ stretching exercises
- ☐ yoga
- ☐ walking (short distances: two miles or less)
- ☐ bicycling (less than 20 minutes)
- ☐ any other aerobic exercise for less than 20 minutes:

_____

_____

_____

- ☐ non-aerobic sports
  - ☐ baseball
  - ☐ bowling
  - ☐ football
  - ☐ golf
  - ☐ volleyball
- ☐ crafts, carpentry
- ☐ gardening (all aspects)
- ☐ work around the house (including normal housework: mowing lawn, raking leaves, vacuuming, cleaning, doing dishes)
- ☐ repair projects (car and home)
- ☐ weight lifting
- ☐ gymnastics

Practice #5

Begin Doing It

Start your exercise program.

First off: Increase your casual exercise as much as you can, and begin your weekly schedule for aerobics. Give yourself two months to adjust to the new schedule. After two months, plan to be following your weekly schedule exactly.

Your long-range goal? To make exercise an integral part of your life, and reap the rewards of increased health, peace, and happiness.

RELAXATION TECHNIQUES

The posture of the body is the posture of the mind made visible.

—*Amrit Desai*

What do you think of when you think of relaxation? Most people think of putting their feet up, lying back, and not doing a thing. But this is not relaxation. Why? When you remain inactive, nervous energy builds. This nervous energy needs to be released through activity, before you can truly relax.

What kind of activity? Physical exercise works well (see preceding section). It discharges tension and leaves you feeling relaxed. Some mental exercises work well also. In the next two sections, you'll learn certain mental practices that will help you reduce tension and manage stress.

In this section, you'll look at physical activities that reduce tension and relax you at the same time, during the activity. These specific techniques not only bring immediate relaxation but leave you feeling relaxed for a long time afterward.

Here are the five most powerful relaxation techniques:

Yoga

Yoga is the most powerful relaxation technique there is. It serves as a complete physical exercise system.

It consists of many different stretching exercises, or poses, which you do in rhythm with your breathing. By breathing as deeply as you can, using your entire lung capacity, and moving as slowly as you breathe, your mind naturally focuses on the harmonious movement of body and breath. During this process, your blood is oxygenated and your heart rate becomes slow and steady. With each pose, you stretch your body to its muscular limit but never exceed this limit. Then, as you hold the pose and breathe as deeply as you can, the muscles you are stretching begin to relax. As they do, you release a tremendous amount of tension from your body.

You'll also notice how different poses massage and tone your internal organs. This helps to heal you. Moreover, the continued practice of yoga makes you feel integrated and at peace with the world.

To learn yoga, take a class with a local certified instructor. Or try any of these books to learn it on your own:

Integral Yoga Hatha by Swami Satchidananda. New York: Holt, Rinehart and Winston, 1970.

Hatha Yoga: Manual I by Samskriti and Veda. Honesdale, PA: Himalayan International Institute, 1986.

Hatha Yoga: The Hidden Language by Swami Sivananda Radha. Palo Alto, CA: Timeless Books, 1989. A workbook by same author and publisher is available: *The Hatha Yoga Workbook.*

Lilias, Yoga and You by Lilias M. Folan. New York: Bantam, 1972.

Light on Yoga (revised edition) by B. K. S. Iyengar. New York: Schocken Books, 1977. (This is highly advanced but perhaps the most definitive book on hatha yoga.)

Or try any one of these videos:

Let's Do Yoga. Mimmie Louis. Redondo Beach, CA: Double Star Productions.

Health, Yoga and Anatomy. Amrita Sandra Mc-Lanahan, MD. Buckingham, VA: Integral Yoga Distribution (Satchidananda Ashram).

Lilias/Alive with Yoga (Volume 1 for Beginners). Lilias M. Folan. Cambridge, MA: Rudra Press.

Deep Rhythmic Breathing

Deep rhythmic breathing relaxes your nervous system and energizes your body. Moreover, once you learn it, you can do it almost anywhere. Here's the basic method:

Lie on your back on the floor. Keep your legs straight or, if it feels more comfortable, pull your feet up until your lower back and the bottoms of your feet rest flat on the floor. Then place your hands on your abdomen, below your rib cage, so you can feel the movement of your diaphragm.

Breathe in slowly, filling the bottom of your lungs

(the area under your hands). Doing this, you should feel your abdomen rising and expanding. Then fill the mid-lungs (lower chest), and feel your rib cage expanding. Complete the inhalation by filling the upper part of your lungs, as you feel your chest opening and rising slightly. Although these three phases seem separate, they occur in one uninterrupted movement, like a wave rising from your abdomen, through your chest.

Now, breathe out slowly, evenly. Empty the bottom of your lungs first, feeling your abdomen flattening. Then empty your mid-lungs and then your upper lungs.

When deep breathing, begin each inhalation and exhalation at the abdomen. With each breath, feel the movement rising up through your chest from the abdomen, as you fill or empty your lungs.

Practice breathing through your nose. Breathe directly into the back of your throat, partially closing your epiglottis, as if snoring faintly. When you breathe into the back of your throat like this, you open the passageways to your lungs. This produces a deep resonant sound by which you can gauge the smoothness and evenness of your breath.

Think of the sound of each breath as a musical note you are holding as long as possible (without running out of breath). This visualization will help you breathe deeply and rhythmically. The deeper and more rhythmic your breath becomes, the more you will relax.

Try taking 20 to 30 breaths each time you practice deep breathing.

You can also learn deep rhythmic breathing by taking a yoga class, because the practice of yoga depends on coordinating bodily movement with the movement of your breath.

After you learn deep rhythmic breathing, you can do it almost anywhere. Even in social situations you can take a few deep breaths and relax, without being conspicuous.

Progressive Relaxation

Progressive relaxation is a way of controlling tension by first creating it, then releasing it. You can do this with your muscles. First you tense a group of muscles and then relax them. By systematically working your way through all the muscle groups in the body, you can relax your entire body. Here's how:

Lie on your back with your arms and legs free. Start with your feet. Tense all the muscles in your feet, then relax them. Repeat two or three times. Now continue the same procedure with each muscle group, in this order: calves, thighs, buttocks, abdomen, chest, back, hands, arms, shoulders, neck, face.

Next, tense all the muscles in your body at once. Then relax. This will help you let go completely. Repeat this process a few times, until your body feels loose and totally relaxed.

Progressive relaxation is a quick way to get rid of anxiety and nervous tension. Try it and see.

Stretching/Warmup Exercises

Traditional American stretching exercises also relax you. Usually done as a warmup, and sometimes a cool-down, to a vigorous workout, these stretching exercises release tension from the muscles. For a good how-to book, try *Stretching* by Bob Anderson (Bolinas, CA: Shelter Publications, 1980).

Sex

Ever think of sex as relaxing? Well, it is . . . but not just any kind of sex.

Relaxation can be achieved after the long-gradual-lovemaking kind of sex. Experts estimate that it takes 30 minutes in the sexual embrace before we experience an actual chemical change inside our bodies. This chemical change has been linked to such positive benefits as the healing of internal organs and the reduction of tension. Complete relaxation washes over lovers after a long embrace.

Important note: Many alcoholic drinkers have health problems pertaining to sex. You may also need to reestablish a positive emotional relationship with your partner. So give your body and your emotions time to heal before trying this technique.

For information on sexual techniques, read:

Sexual Secrets by Nik Douglas and Penny Slinger. New York: Destiny Books, 1979.

The Tao of Love and Sex by Jolan Chang. London: Wildwood House, 1977.

The Art of Sexual Ecstasy by Margo Annand. Los Angeles: Tarcher, 1989.

The Joy of Sex by Alex Comfort. New York: Simon & Schuster, 1972.

ESO: Extended Sexual Orgasm by Alan and Donna Bauer. New York: Warner Books, 1983.

Checklist #3

Relaxers: What Works Best for You?

Instructions: Try all the relaxation techniques just described. Then select the two or three that work best for you. Check them on the list below and begin using them regularly.

☐   yoga
☐   deep rhythmic breathing
☐   progressive relaxation
☐   stretching/warmup exercises
☐   sex

ASSERTIVENESS TRAINING

When dealing with other people, do you remain on an even keel? Most people don't. We tend to overreact or underreact, at least some of the time. What happens when we behave this way? Our stress level increases.

At one extreme, you may blow up too often, yelling or screaming or getting hostile with others.

At the other extreme, you may let other people run over you too often. You may become silent or overly agreeable, or simply let other people get their way too often.

When you act too much at either extreme, tension builds and your relationships will seem distorted or incomplete. In one case, you force too much of yourself on others. In the other case, you give too much of yourself up.

But there is a middle ground. Your behavior in your relationships can be both socially appropriate and emotionally fulfilling. This middle ground is like

Baby Bear's porridge in the story of the three bears: it's not too hot, not too cold, but just right.

This middle ground is called assertive behavior; the extreme stances just described are called, respectively, aggressive and passive behavior. The more you act from the middle ground in your relationships, the better you will feel. Assertive behavior means sticking up for your rights and protecting your needs, without overdoing it. It means you don't let others push you around, nor do you push others around to get your own way. Let's look at some examples.

Situation: You're waiting in a long line at the grocery store or the movies. Someone butts in line ahead of you.

Aggressive response: You get mad and start yelling, "Hey you . . . get out of here! Get back to the end of the line where you belong!" After an incident like this, your anger and tension stay high for a long time.

Passive response: You don't say a thing. You get mad but you keep it inside. Soon you get mad at yourself for being such a pushover, for letting people get away with such things. Your tension and internal stress remain high for quite a long time after the incident.

Assertive response: You go up to the person and say, in a normal tone, "I know you must be in a hurry, but we've all been waiting for a long time before you got here. Please go to the end of the line and wait your turn like everyone else." With this response, you do something to solve a problem. Even if the person wants to argue, when you remain levelheaded that person will look like a fool.

You will confront numerous situations every day that call for assertive behavior. A cashier may short-change you, a waiter may bring you the wrong order, someone may jump in the door of the taxi you just hailed. These situations happen among strangers, but most problems with behavior transpire among friends, especially intimate friends. Among close friends, one person may yell to get her way, another person may passively give in all the time. This is common. Yet relationships like these remain immature. They do not grow, because they lack fairness. Partners in these relationships bully the other or allow themselves to be bullied. In either case the relationship feels incomplete.

Which kind of person are you? Are you aggressive or passive? How can you become assertive? Here are some books that will help:

> *When I Say No I Feel Guilty* by Manuel J. Smith, Ph.D. New York: Bantam, 1975.

> *Your Perfect Right: A Guide to Assertive Living* by Robert Alberti, Ph.D., and Michael L. Emmons, Ph.D. San Luis Obispo, CA: Impact Publishers, 1990.

Now try Practice #6.

Practice #6

Assertive Responses:
How to Remain Centered

Instructions: Write assertive responses to the following situations. Practice them to yourself. Then practice using these responses when confronted by the situations.

Neighbor playing music too loud.
Your assertive response: _____

_____

_____

_____

You are taking a friend to a meeting. Yet the friend keeps puttering around for a half-hour so that you will arrive late.
Your assertive response: _____

_____

_____

_____

After you have changed to a healthy diet, a friend of yours offers you candy or cookies.
Your assertive response: _____

_____

_____

_____

After you have quit drinking, an old friend tries to get you to drink, saying, "C'mon, just one or two won't hurt. I'll buy."
Your assertive response: _____

_____

_____

_____

What other situation can you think of?
Situation: _____

_____

_____

_____

Your assertive response: _____

_____

_____

_____

Remember, assertiveness is another way to reduce your stress. And clearly, the less stressed you feel, the less you will want to drink.

STRESS MANAGEMENT
AND COPING TECHNIQUES

You have just learned how exercise, relaxation techniques, and assertiveness skills can help reduce stress. Here are 22 other effective techniques. Most of them are simple mental exercises anyone can use with a little practice.

Checklist #4

22 Surefire Stress Reducers

Instructions: Go over the list and get a feel for the various coping skills. Which do you like the most? Choose seven or more of these alternatives—the ones you think would work for you. Then, whenever you feel stressed, do one or more of the techniques you have selected.

☐ *Imagine a pleasant moment.* Maybe you concentrate too much on what goes wrong in your life. Now concentrate on what has gone right. Think of at least one pleasant moment you experienced in the past week. What were your feelings? How did it happen? Re-create the moment in your mind as fully as you can. Remember it. Dwell on it. Enjoy the utter happiness of that moment once again.

☐ *Desensitize stressful moments.* If you do concentrate too much on what goes wrong, take a closer look now at what goes wrong. Usually the trouble is not so much what has happened as your reaction to it. Visualize something that has gone wrong for you. What was it? Now visualize yourself responding in a positive way to the same situation. Imagine yourself making this positive response the next time the situation arises. Imagine this positive outcome over and over for 10 to 15 minutes. You'll be surprised how much better you'll feel about the situation and how much better you'll deal with the same situation in the future.

☐ *Live in the moment.* Instead of remembering a pleasant moment from the past, create a pleasant moment now. Live it fully. Concentrate all your attention on a beautiful object, such as a flower or a candle flame. Drop all thoughts. Don't try to label or describe the beauty, but simply experience it in silence. Allow the pleasant sensations to wash over you, and become one with the object of your attention.

☐ *Transcendental meditation.* Silently or out loud, repeat to yourself a sound, a word, or a phrase, over and over, in rhythmic cadence, for 15 to 20 minutes. Some sounds you can use: Om, Aum, Hum, Mmmm. Some words: One, God, Love, Sun. Some phrases: Peace on Earth, All Is One, On and On, World Without End. It helps if you synchronize the sound with your breathing. Why does this practice work? It helps you focus your mind and become centered.

☐ *Silent meditation.* Sit comfortably, preferably in a yoga sitting position. Now focus on your breath. Consider this: Your breath is your entire life. Oxygen is food. Without oxygen from breathing, you would die. As you breathe, imagine yourself taking nourishment into all the cells of your body. Breathe deeply and slowly, paying attention to each breath. Gradually you'll feel the life you gain from breathing, and with it, a deep sense of gratitude.

☐ *Take a vacation.* Get away from it all. Go to the shore, the mountains, anywhere, as long as it offers you a fresh environment. Best bet: Plan a vacation at a health spa and revitalize yourself while you enjoy the new surroundings.

☐ *Read a book.* Pick your favorite kind of reading material. Kick back and get into it. Two birds with one stone? Read a self-help book on how to reduce stress.

☐ *Leave work at work.* Don't bring work home with you. Don't think about work once you're at home. It's fine to put in extra hours if it doesn't stress you out. But remember to cut back as soon as you feel strain, tension, or fatigue. Look at it this way: If you work eight hours a day and sleep eight hours a day, that leaves you eight hours to yourself. Use them for yourself. Plan leisure activities you like to do . . . and do them.

☐ *Solve problems.* If something's bothering you, it's important to identify the problem. Take time to understand the problem—view it from all sides—then solve it. You can solve your own problems or solve any kind of problems you choose. Some people find it relaxing to discover the solutions to various kinds of puzzles and math problems.

☐ *Play with a pet.* Research shows that playing with a pet lowers blood pressure and heart rate. In other words, it relaxes you. Even more interesting, your pet doesn't have to be a "pettable" pet. Watching fish in an aquarium has been shown to have the same soothing effects.

☐ *Sing.* Singing is one of the most calming things you can do. When very happy, you can sing for joy. When sad, you can sing the blues. Singing expresses feeling. By singing, you let your feelings out, releasing your emotions to the world. So whether it's with a group of friends or in the shower stall, belt out a tune and light up your life with song.

☐ *Enjoy plants.* Plants bring peaceful feelings. From indoor potted varieties to flower beds to outdoor vegetable gardens, working with plants can be most relaxing. Just looking at plants, or having plants near you, brings a feeling of calm. Extra benefits: Indoor plants brighten your home and freshen the air; flower beds and shrubs beautify your grounds; vegetable gardens offer peaceful food for a peaceful table. So tend a garden, pot a plant, sow a seed, or prune a bush.

☐ *Get into cooking.* It's not for everyone, but many people can become totally involved in cooking. Creating a meal can be pleasurable and extremely relaxing. If you're one who can let your cares float away in the kitchen, go for it—bake, broil, chop, sauté, and stir-fry away.

☐ *Bathe yourself.* Treat yourself to a long, relaxing bath. In the perfect warm-hot water, cares dissolve and tension melts away. Before entering the peaceful waters of your tub, close the bathroom door, lock it, and close your mind to everything outside the room. If you like, add some herbal essence or special fragrance to enhance the effect.

☐ *Take a class on stress management.* Here's a good way to learn more about reducing your stress. You will gain many pointers not covered in this book and, in the group, you can share your experiences with others.

☐ *Walk away.* A simple technique: When frustrated with something or someone, walk away. Do not return until you cool down.

☐ *Do nothing.* This option is more like meditation. Do nothing—absolutely nothing. Look at a blank wall. Keep your mind blank. Don't allow a single thought to form. Fight every thought as if it were an intrusion into your imperturbable silence. Do this for 15 to 20 minutes and you'll feel incredibly refreshed.

☐ *Groan.* Sound peculiar? Well, it's not. Groaning helps our bodies handle pain. When you hurt yourself physically—even just stubbing your toe—notice how groaning relieves some of the pain. Groan for a few minutes right now. Notice how it reduces tension. Try it when you want to relax.

☐ *Cry.* This is the ultimate stress reducer. Since the beginning of time, crying has helped the body get rid of inner toxins and release emotional pain. It's the natural response to stress and suffering. Cry whenever you feel the need.

☐ *Talk it out.* If some other person is bothering you, talk it out. Work together with that person to find a common solution. If you can't work with that person to find a solution, talk with someone else. Talking about your problems gets them out in the open and relieves you of most of the stress.

☐ *Get lost in a fun activity.* When disturbed by outside stress, do some activity that you love to do. Dive into your favorite, most fun-filled pastime. Dissolve tension with excitement, gaiety, amusement.

☐   *Be thankful.* Show gratitude for anything. Gratitude is
the most calming emotion there is. Take time to feel
thoroughly thankful for a meal . . . a friend . . . a family member . . . your own health . . . your ability to
change something in your life. Be thankful for life itself.

FRIENDSHIP

*Friendship is a strong and habitual inclination
in two persons to promote the good and happiness of one another.*
—Eustace Budgell

There's hardly anything in this world more precious
than a friend. A friend can listen to your troubles and
help you solve them. Or, if you cannot solve your
troubles, a friend will help you feel at peace.

Friendship helps you feel strong inside. Even
when everything around you seems gloomy, friendship feels warm. Friendship feels solid. It's one of life's
primary needs to know that someone cares for you.

What is a friend? Someone you feel comfortable
with. Someone you can tell anything—and everything—about yourself.

Good friends are truthful. They won't lie to you.
Perhaps more important, good friends won't let you
lie to them.

With a friend, you can talk about your miseries,
your shattered dreams, and as you talk, these problems simply drift away. Anger becomes sympathy, re-
sentment turns to forgiveness, fear converts to love
when talking to a friend. Indeed, your best therapist is
a good friend.

Practice #7

Find One Good Friend

Instructions: Because friendship is so important to your emotional strength, be sure to have at least one good friend when you quit drinking. This friend may drink, but be sure that he or she is not an alcoholic.

Most alcoholics have two sets of friends, one set that's alcoholic and one that's not. When you quit drinking, hang out with your nonalcoholic friends. Choose your best friend from that group and begin seeing that person more often.

Why is this so important? Active alcoholics normally associate with other alcoholics and they support each other with reasons to keep drinking. Misery loves company.

Yet abruptly changing friends often causes its own problems. That's why it's best to take your time with it. New friends will soon appear. Just keep working toward strong, positive friendships, and don't let old, negative friendships drag you down. Remain steadfast and open with everyone.

Who is your best friend? Sometimes the person you think is your best friend really is not. When you choose a friend, make sure you can answer yes to all these questions:

☐ Can I talk confidentially about anything and everything with this person?

☐ Can this person help me understand my feelings without persuading me to act in a certain way?

☐ Will this person help me make my own decisions?

☐ Do I feel this person is on my side?

☐ Can we laugh at things together?

☐ Do we enjoy each other's company?

☐ Do I feel this friendship will endure through time, through difficult periods as well as good periods?

Can a lover be a best friend? Yes.

Can a therapist be a best friend? Yes.

If you can't find a best friend among the friends you have, you may find a best friend in your lover—if he or she meets the above criteria. But if you cannot find anyone at this time to be your best friend, get a therapist. Make sure you can answer yes to all the above questions when evaluating your therapist too. Keep looking until you find the therapist that's right for you.

Now, in order to complete this worksheet, list the one person who will be your best friend. Write his or her name here: _____

If you have a backup best friend (or therapist), write

that person's name here: _____

Of course, be sure to rely on your best friend or backup whenever you feel in need of emotional support.

CHAPTER 8

Thirty Additional Ways to Renew Yourself

The art of life lies in a constant readjustment to our surroundings.

—Okakura Kakuzo

U sing all that you've learned so far, imagine you were cooking up a cure for alcoholism. Diet would be the main ingredient. Then you'd add exercise and relaxation techniques, assertiveness, coping, and friendship skills. Now—just before stirring—it's time to add some spices, to make the dish complete.

In this chapter, you'll find the spices: 30 effective methods of healing. Used liberally with the main ingredients, these methods will help cure you of the problems caused by alcohol. They will help heal your body, build your emotional strength, and relax you.

So add some zest to your life. Add some zip. Plan to use at least five or six of these methods in your program for quitting drinking. You'll have more control over your life and be assured of greater success.

After you read about these methods and consider which ones you'd like to do, in Worksheet #7 you can select the ones you will do.

THE AMAZING SUCCESS OF ACUPUNCTURE

This relatively new method for treating alcoholism and drug addiction increases individual success rates so dramatically, it appears to act as a cure in itself.

Acupuncture is not new, of course. Refined and cultivated for about 3,000 years in the Far East, this proven method is finally gaining widespread acceptance in the United States.

What is acupuncture? It involves rechanneling the energy of the body for the purpose of healing. You can receive treatments for almost any kind of ailment, including simple pain. The treatment for alcohol withdrawal involves placing five very thin, short needles on outer ear points for 30 to 45 minutes. This treatment is so easy, it can be done in a waiting room, on a walk-in basis.

How does it work? Stimulating these points on the outer ear creates an energy exchange with the brain, causing it to automatically produce endorphins. Instantly, you experience a natural high— with no drugs, no alcohol. So not only is the treatment completely painless, it generates feelings of total euphoria. Eighty percent of individuals receiving this treatment report an improvement in how they feel. (Among the remaining 20%, it should be noted that some of them felt some pain from the needles.)

Current studies on acupuncture show 50%–60% success rates. "Success" in these studies means the clients did not resume drinking during the first six-month period of treatment. Although longer-term studies are needed, this still compares very favorably with AA's 12%–25% success rate over a three-year period. Ideally, long-term results would show a decrease in the need for acupuncture treatment as the brain regained control of its own endorphin production.

Check your area for acupuncture clinics or holistic health centers. Also consult alcohol and drug treatment centers. Many now offer acupuncture on an outpatient basis.

Acupressure. Acupressure attempts the same results without the needles, by applying pressure through finger massage and squeezing. It is an effective treatment, though not as powerful as acupuncture. You may prefer an acupressure massage, called shiatsu, to relax the whole body. (For information on acupressure and massage, see the next section.)

Another Variation: CES. CES stands for cranial electro-stimulation (it's also known as NET, which is short for neuro-electric therapy). For CES, adhesive electrodes are attached to ear points (behind the ear so as not to be too visible), and wires connect to a stimulator worn on a belt or put in a pocket. It has a button that can send a mild current to the ear points. This current causes stimulation similar to the acupuncture needles that prompts the brain to produce endorphins. The interesting plus about CES is that you can get the stimulation anytime you need it. If you feel a little down, just press a button.

For specific information on CES/NET, try:

Hooked! NET: The New Approach to Drug Cure by Meg Patterson, MBE, MBChB, FRCSE. London: Faber and Faber, 1986.

For your own CES machine, try:

Tools for Exploration 800-456-9887 for catalog

Inner Quest 800-628-MIND for catalog

MASSAGE ... FOR HEALTH AND RELAXATION

When you bang into something and hurt yourself, what's the first thing you do? Rub the sore spot. And for good reason. Rubbing soothes the area and diminishes the pain.

A massage is nothing more than a good rub—to soothe the entire body. It helps reduce tension, release stress, and dissolve your aches and pains. In addition, many professionals claim a great amount of healing power for various types of massage.

It's one thing to exchange massages with loved ones or friends. You may want to do that. But also be sure to try a few sessions with one or more local professionals. You'll be amazed at the incredible transformation you can achieve at the hands of a professional.

When seeking a professional massage, you may find the following descriptions helpful:

Acupressure/Shiatsu. Based on the acupuncture medical model for improving energy flow in the body, it involves deep pressing with fingers, knuckles, and thumbs. It's warming, increases circulation, relieves tension, and improves healing of internal organs.

Swedish Massage. Softer than acupressure, this method is characterized by long smooth strokes, usually with the open hand. Relaxing and warming, it releases muscle tension.

Sports Massage. This more active kind of rubbing with the open hand involves some percussion, or drumming, on the body with hands. It's good for releasing muscle tension, including muscle cramps, and for increasing circulation.

Rolfing. Perhaps the most intense and comprehensive of all massages (ten sessions to "complete the course"), this method, named for its inventor, Ida Rolf, involves everything from soft, smooth touch to hard, almost painful, kneading of deep tissue. It is said to "realign" the body, balance the mind, correct internal energies, and heal bodily organs. Many prominent people have been Rolfed and give glowing testimonials.

For more information on various alternatives, write to:

Associated Bodywork & Massage Professionals
PO Box 1869
Evergreen, CO 80439

American Massage Therapy Association
820 Davis Street, Suite 100,
Evanston, IL 60201

BIOFEEDBACK

When you feel good, your brain produces alpha waves. Exercise, meditation, restful sleep, and creative activity all stimulate the production of alpha waves. When the alpha waves flow, your mind is relaxed.

The original biofeedback machines measured alpha waves; and when the brain emitted a certain level of alpha, the machine gave a signal. With this process people learned how to increase their own alpha output. More important, once they had learned it and practiced it, they didn't need the equipment anymore. They could go into "alpha state" at will, almost any time of the day, whenever they needed to relax.

Now biofeedback machines can help you control many of the so-called involuntary bodily functions. For instance, you can learn to raise or lower your heart rate at will. You can learn to reduce muscle tension, body temperature, and nervousness. All of these learned responses are surefire ways to decrease stress and increase your feelings of relaxation.

To get yourself connected to a biofeedback machine, try your local mental health clinic or a psychotherapist. Or to buy your own, try Tools for Exploration, 800-456-9887, or Inner Quest 800-628-MIND.

BODYWORK/BODY MOVEMENT

You have studied many forms of bodywork already: various exercises, yoga, stretching, and so on. A list of some additional forms follows. Each can help heal you and reduce your stress.

Tai chi. A beautiful form of bodily motion with exercises based on energy balancing, it is said to have internal healing power.

Martial arts. Kung fu, karate, jujitsu, akido. Exercises facilitate strength, coordination, and movement.

Alexander Technique. Involves methods for body balancing and working with spinal alignment in your normal everyday activity.

Feldenkrais method. A series of "body lessons" increase individuals' awareness of inner movement, flexibility, and coordination.

Ohashiatsu. Teaches you to balance internal energies through movements and self-massage.

And many, many more: for instance, Rubenfeld Synergy, Trager Mind-Body Integration, polarity therapy, Neo-Reichian/bioenergetics. All of these use various combinations of methods to help you balance your energy, heal internal organs, and relax.

These methods work with varying degrees of effectiveness for different individuals. Experiment to find which work best for you.

Where can you find listings? Check any "new age" directory in your area, as well as alternative newspapers and magazines. If you have a holistic health center nearby, call and ask for information on what they offer.

HYPNOSIS

Through the power of suggestion, a hypnotist can plant a thought in your mind that you'll remember after the session. This can help you in two ways. The hypnotist can coax you to feel more relaxed in certain situations that would normally bother you. And the hypnotist can create powerful built-in reminders to help you control your desire to drink.

Over the past few decades, hypnotists have

achieved great success in these two areas. Unfortunately, hypnosis doesn't work for everyone. Only about half of the population can be hypnotized.

That means you have a 50/50 chance it could work for you. So if you're interested, check it out.

AUTOGENIC TRAINING/SELF-HYPNOSIS

Research shows that individuals can learn to relax by lying comfortably with eyes closed and repeating certain key phrases to themselves. This is called autogenic training or self-hypnosis. Sample phrases include: "My breath is calm and regular." "My heartbeat feels slow and certain." "My body feels heavy." "I feel warm all over." "My nerves will settle now." And so on.

A trained therapist can help you get started, then you can do it on your own. Or you can just start by doing it on your own—it's not that hard. (By the way, autogenic training coupled with biofeedback has been shown to be doubly effective. If you choose one, you may want to add the other.)

VISUALIZATION

Please take a moment to relax. Now imagine yourself sucking on a lemon. Imagine the tart taste of lemon juice filling your mouth. Imagine it on your tongue. Now stop the image and check yourself. Your mouth is slightly puckered and loaded with saliva. Why? Your imagination is so powerful that it can actually change what happens to you physically.

To be sure, whatever you imagine about yourself can dramatically change your life. Studies show that when you're sick and you imagine yourself healing the ailment, you have a much better chance of getting well. These studies have noted improved success with a variety of ailments, physical problems, and diseases, including cancer.

How can you use this technique when you quit drinking? After you quit the alcohol, visualize yourself getting well. Visualize your body healing the many physical ailments alcohol has caused. Visualize yourself in the image of health.

Imagine a war inside. Imagine yourself winning. Over and over, imagine yourself winning, and gaining the reward of good health.

Here's yet another way to use visualization: Imagine yourself resisting the temptation to drink. Imagine yourself saying (inside yourself), "I don't need it anymore. I've outgrown it. I prefer to be healthy now. I want to be free. It's time now for me to grow up." Imagine yourself going through a heroic transformation. Visualize yourself getting better and better.

You can use visualization another way too. Imagine yourself in a situation where someone, maybe an old friend, is coaxing you to drink. Imagine yourself refusing. Imagine yourself refusing politely yet firmly. Imagine exactly what you'll say to the person. Something like: "No thanks, I've quit for health reasons. Alcohol nearly killed me, and I can't drink anymore." Practice saying your reason over and over.

One other way you can use visualization: Whenever you think about drinking, imagine your worst drunk. Remember it completely. Maybe you nearly died or felt like you could have died. Maybe you embarrassed yourself beyond belief, made a mistake that cost you thousands of dollars (wrecked automobiles, legal fees, and so on), or seriously hurt someone. Now imagine yourself avoiding these kinds of problems completely. Imagine becoming proud of yourself for doing well in life. Imagine all this as one of your main reasons to avoid alcohol.

AFFIRMATIONS

This technique combines some elements of both self-hypnosis and visualization. An affirmation is a positive statement about yourself that you repeat over and over again, until your subconscious gets the message. Hers's a way to say yes to yourself—a way to change and to help yourself grow.

Here's the technique: Choose your affirmation and repeat it over and over. Repeat it silently to yourself. Repeat it out loud whenever you can. Also write it. Write the entire affirmation over and over, 20 to 30 times at a sitting. Do this at least once a day.

To get you started, here are some ideas for affirmations. You can change the words of any affirmation to make it sound more like you. Select one or two affirmations and keep working with them until you feel yourself changing.

To help with quitting

My body keeps regaining health.

I'm becoming strong.

I envision myself thinking clearly now.

I see myself in control of my thoughts and actions.

I feel comfortable in my body.

I choose not to drink.

I will avoid alcohol . . . it has been ruining my life.

I want to be healthy.

I will find greater happiness.

My body radiates health.

My body radiates happiness.

Now I choose to grow.

Now I will mature.

Now I'm in control.

I'm free to be myself.

To handle guilt over past actions

I forgive myself for mistakes I've made.

I forgive myself for hurting myself.

I can't change the past. It's done and gone. But I
will change the future.

From Sondra Ray's book, *Loving Relationships*:

I forgive myself for hurting others.

I forgive myself for struggling in life.

I forgive others for hurting me.

I am innocent. I am a child of God. All my desires
are holy and they always have been.

You can find many other affirmations—and ways
to use them—in *Loving Relationships* by Sondra Ray.
I recommend this book.

SUBLIMINAL SUGGESTION

Today, there are many audio and video tapes that
make use of "subliminal suggestion." These tapes
promise to help you change something about yourself.
Some of the subjects: "How to Quit Drinking," "How
to Quit Smoking," "How to Relax."

How do they work? The audiotapes have a
soundtrack of music or ocean waves, and a secondary

inaudible soundtrack which is nevertheless perceived by your subconscious mind. The videotapes present some pleasant visual scene with visual messages interspersed at 1/46 second—too fast for your eye to see, yet perceptible to your subconscious. At the same time, the video's soundtrack is embedded with subliminal vocal messages.

These messages are much like the affirmations just described. Here's a sampling of messages from three different subliminal tapes on quitting drinking.

From Gateways Institute, Ojai, CA:

I am free of dependency on alcohol.

I dislike alcohol.

I refuse alcoholic drinks offered to me.

From Success Education Institute International, San Diego, CA:

I do not drink alcohol.

Alcohol is poison for me.

I like having self-control.

I take life one day at a time.

I am a winner today and every day.

From Mind Communications, Inc., Grand Rapids, MI:

I love my body.

Drugs are dumb.

Alcohol is poison.

Alcohol hurts me.

I am good to me.

You can find other tapes with other variations.

When you select a subliminal tape, make sure its messages match your feelings. For instance, if you don't like the phrase "I take life one day at a time," the second tape above will not be good for you.

Subliminal tapes do not work for everyone. In fact, when measured scientifically, visualization and affirmation techniques show higher success rates. But you may want to try them all to see what works best for you.

A CLINIC OR A LIVE-IN PROGRAM

Ever think of taking some time off and going somewhere for intensive treatment? It might be just what you need. The right treatment center, clinic, or health resort can greatly improve your chances for success.

Why? Because it gives you an opportunity to reorganize yourself in a safe environment. At your own pace, you can change your ways. Moreover, getting away from the environment you associate with your habits and problems, and from the daily struggle of coping, can do wonders.

Does this sound like it could be for you? If so, plan to go to a clinic or enter a live-in program soon after you have quit drinking. Probably the best time for this is immediately after detox. In fact, many alcohol treatment facilities combine detox with an ongoing program. The detox phase may take 4 to 7 days, and a live-in phase may take another 7 to 25 days or more. A clinic may keep you on an outpatient basis for as long as a year or even longer.

Many different types of clinics and live-in programs, offering a wide variety of services, are available. And keep in mind that most, but not all, treatment programs are covered by medical insurance.

What kind of services can you expect?

The majority of alcohol treatment centers and clinics base their approach on the "Minnesota model" developed in Hazelden in the 1950s. These centers offer primarily three things: psychotherapy, education, and AA. Studies at these centers have shown their three-year success rate to be fairly low (between 5% and 25%).

But a new kind of center, started in the 1980s, offers a broader approach to recovery, called a whole-person approach. These centers treat all aspects of the individual: the physical, the emotional, the mental, and the spiritual. The key addition here is the physical. These new centers address physical healing and biochemical repair of the individual. Techniques include nutritional therapy, dietary counseling, exercise, stress reduction techniques, and relaxation skills.

And of course when individuals reduce their physical stress, they can achieve greater healing mentally, emotionally, and spiritually as well. This "overall healing" shows in the success rates of centers offering a whole-person approach. Studies reveal that one-, two-, and three-year success rates for these centers range from 50% to 90%.

Among these centers, most still incorporate AA as part of their overall program. Some in fact require that you attend AA, yet other centers make it optional, and some centers have dropped AA altogether. Here is a list of centers that offer a whole-person approach to recovery. (Note: all of these have a strong component for physical healing, including stress reduction, exercise, and relaxation techniques, and most have some kind of plan for dietary intervention as well.)

Comprehensive Medical Care
Amityville, NY
516-598-2960

- Outpatient
- Well-balanced whole-person approach
- Very strong dietary component
- AA is optional
- One-year success rate: 60.4%

Betty Ford Center
Rancho Mirage, CA
800-392-7540 (in CA)
800-854-9211 (out of state)

- Inpatient and outpatient
- Registered dietician on staff
- Very strong on AA
- One-year success rate: 65%

Forest Hospital Rational Recovery Program
Des Plaines, IL
708-635-4100

- Inpatient and outpatient
- Well-balanced whole-person approach
- Nutrition therapy
- AA is not offered—this is a complete alternative approach

Greenleaf Health Systems
Chattanooga, TN (headquarters)
615-870-5110

- Numerous facilities
- Inpatient and outpatient
- Offers nutritional counseling
- AA recommended

Hampstead Hospital Rational Recovery Program
Hampstead, NH
603-329-5311

- Inpatient and outpatient
- AA is not offered—this is a complete alternative approach

Health Recovery Center
Minneapolis, MN
612-827-7800

- Outpatient
- Well-balanced whole-person approach
- Very strong dietary component
- AA is optional
- One-year success rate: 75%

Merritt Peralta Institute
Oakland, CA
510-652-7000

- Inpatient and outpatient
- Offers nutrition information
- AA recommended

Milam Recovery Programs
Seattle, WA (headquarters)
206-241-0890
800-544-1211

- Three centers in Washington
- Inpatient and outpatient
- Nutritional therapy and training
- AA is recommended

Parc Place
Phoenix, AZ
602-840-4774

- For adolescents
- Inpatient and outpatient
- Addresses dietary concerns
- AA is recommended
- Two-year success rate: 76%

Parkside Programs
Park Ridge, IL (headquarters)
708-698-4700
800-PARKSIDE

- 43 inpatient and 23 outpatient facilities in 18 states
- Programs for adults and adolescents
- Addresses nutritional issues
- Very strong on AA
- Two-year success rate, adults: 81.9% (the adolescent recovery rate was significantly less)

The Phoenix Center
St Louis, MO
314-781-0018
Also: Kansas City, MO
816-353-7400

- Outpatient
- AA is not offered

Pride Institute
Eden Prarie, MN
800-54-PRIDE

- For gay men, lesbians, and bisexuals
- Inpatient and outpatient
- Nutritious diet
- AA recommended
- 14-month success rate: 74%

Recovery Systems
Mill Valley, CA
415-383-3611

- Outpatient
- Well-balanced whole-person approach
- Very strong dietary component
- AA is optional

Rational Recovery–Residential
Lotus, CA
916-621-2667

- Inpatient (the Rational Recovery residential Program at its home office)
- AA is not offered—this is a complete alternative approach

3HO Super Health
Tucson, AZ
602-749-0404

- Inpatient
- Well-balanced whole-person approach
- AA is optional
- Three year success rate: 76%

Valley Hope Association
Norton, KS (headquarters)
913-877-5111
800-654-0486

- 12 inpatient and 5 outpatient centers in seven states
- Nutritional counseling
- Recommends AA
- "Fly to Recovery" program from anywhere in United States
- 11 of the top 100 centers in the book *The 100 Best Treatment Centers for Alcoholism and Drug Abuse* are Valley Hope centers.

In Canada, contact:

Canadian Centre on Substance Abuse/National Clearinghouse on Substance Abuse
112 Kent Way, Suite 480
Ottawa, Ontario K1P 5P2
613-235-4048

- Ask for the address of your provincial center that can give you a list of treatment facilities in your province.

Of course, for healing purposes, don't feel limited to alcohol rehabilitation centers. You can find many different kinds of health resorts and spiritual retreats across the country. Once you complete detox, you can choose any of these that suits you.

The recent *New Age Sourcebook*, from the editors of the *New Age Journal*, lists over 35 holistic health resorts and retreats. Of course, AA is not spoken at these centers, yet their programs can help renew you. Here are a few that have specialized programs for those recovering from addictions:

Himalayan Institute
Honesdale, PA
800-822-4547
"Addictions Recovery" (duration: a minimum of four weeks; recommended: three months).

Kripalu Center
Lenox, MA
413-448-3400
Seven-day program: "The Yoga of Recovery." (Participants must have at least two years of continuous sobriety.)

Omega Institute
Rhinebeck, NY
914-266-4301
Various programs and workshops each summer (Ask for summer catalog.)

Satchidananda Ashram
Buckingham, VA
804-969-3121
"Breaking Free: Overcoming Addictions Through Yoga," a three-day intensive.

SOLITUDE AND SELF-REFLECTION

How do you feel about being alone? Perhaps you like it. Perhaps you find you gain strength whenever you take an hour or two to be completely by yourself.

If so, you've got plenty of company. Many people need to make time for themselves, away from the crowd, to sort things out alone.

Solitude is one of life's most rewarding experiences. It gives you a chance to examine yourself and make plans for self-renewal. It can be a time for artistic creation, self-reflection, resolution, or inner peace.

Use your solitude to your advantage and it will help renew you.

A precaution: You must be relaxed. If you spend your time alone nervously worrying about yourself, it will do no good. Best bet: If you feel nervous or anxious, take care of that first. Then your solitude will be calming and your self-reflection will bring strength.

HEALING WITH LAUGHTER

Ho, ho, ho, ha, ha, hee, hee, hee. Laugh right now. Notice how it calms you? A hearty laugh not only calms the body but helps it heal.

Some studies have shown that laughter, like exercise, produces endorphins, the body's natural tranquilizers. Other studies have found that laughter stimulates the immune system by increasing antibodies and lowering cortisol. That means laughter promotes physical healing and greater strength against disease.

So laugh it up. Enjoy something funny. Give a great guffaw. Chuckle, bellow, hahaha.

Here are some suggestions:

- Watch comedians or a funny movie on TV.
- Go to comedy clubs.
- Read the comics.
- Hang around funny people: jokesters, pranksters, and so on.
- Go to a circus to see the clowns (or hire a clown to come to your home for birthday parties).
- Read a funny book: a joke book or a humorous novel.
- Look for more humor in yourself, in every little thing you do.
- Act silly . . . clown around whenever you can.
- Look for more humor in the universe. Meditate on this. Our universe is really a very funny place, you know.

TURN OFF YOUR TV

TV increases your nervous energy in two ways. First, it keeps you inactive, sitting in front of the set. Second, it blasts your body with a constant barrage of electrons.

How does TV work? An electron gun shoots electrons at the screen. This produces the image. But the electrons don't stop at the screen. They come right through the screen and enter the human body. This "electron bath" can be very dangerous. Electrons, which are negatively charged electrical particles, can wreak havoc on your nervous system. Why? Your nervous system depends on a balance of positive and negative charges.

Laboratory rats placed in front of a color TV

showed extreme hyperactivity for the first ten days to a month. Their behavior during this time was nervous, restless, even aggressive and hostile. Then the animals began to show fatigue. They became so lethargic they needed a push just to get them to move around the cage. Other studies have found that if two color TV sets are aimed at young rats, many of them die. The reason? Autopsies indicate severe brain tissue damage.

Not only does TV make you nervous and interfere with mental functioning, it takes precious time that you could be using to do something positive for yourself. For instance, you could be exercising—something that actually reduces depression and fatigue. You could be reading an important book, taking a night class, building something, creating something, or having fun.

Now let's back up for a minute. Some TV shows may be exceptions. You may actually gain some benefits from:

- Watching educational programming that can help you learn something important.
- Watching TV exercise programs (or exercise videotapes) *while doing the exercises.*
- Watching a show that makes you laugh—for instance, a comedy routine or some really hilarious show (a sitcom that forces you to sit through a half-hour of drudgery for two or three laughs is not worth it).

So . . . what to do? Cut out almost all TV. Allow yourself eight to ten hours a week, maximum. This includes anything you watch on videotape as well.

The less TV the better. How will you do it? Plan your week ahead of time. For instance, you may want to watch three or four shows during the week and a movie or sporting event on the weekend. Make up your mind. If this is your plan, stick to it—don't watch any more TV that week.

FASTING

Here's a healing method as old as the human race itself. Animals use it regularly. When sick, animals will naturally stop eating for a while until they get better. Humans have the same instinct. In all cultures, throughout history, we have used fasting as a primary method of healing.

But fasting does more than just heal the body. It can clear your thoughts and illuminate your mind. The world's greatest spiritual leaders have all used fasting as a means to inner enlightenment—Jesus, Buddha, Muhammad, Gandhi, to name just a few.

How does fasting help? It rids the body of toxins, thus leading the way to better health. Routinely the body stores toxins and unwanted chemical buildup in the body fat. A fast breaks down the body fat, thereby releasing the toxins into the bloodstream. The body then excretes the toxins through normal channels of elimination.

There are many kinds of fasts and methods of fasting. Here's a brief overview:

- *Normal daily fasting.* Go about 12 hours without food every day, say from 7 in the evening to 7 the next morning. This gives the body time to get rid of some unwanted chemical buildup and metabolic debris. You break fast with breakfast.

- *Only two meals a day.* One at 3 P.M., one at 7 P.M. This kind of fast gives the body an even longer break.

- *One or two full days (or more).* This can help clear the body of a great amount of excess junk. After two full days, you begin to get into spiritual fasting. However, if you plan to go more than two days, it's best to get supervision. Many health resorts offer supervised fasting.

- *Water fast.* You need to drink lots of liquids on a fast. If you're a purist, you might drink only water.

- *Juice fast.* The liquid of choice: fresh-squeezed natural organic juices. This is probably the best liquid for fasting, since the alkalizing effects of the juice offset the acid-forming effects of toxins being released into the bloodstream. Vegetable broth may also be used with just about the same effects as juice.

Note: Do not attempt to fast if you are more than ten pounds underweight, if you have any serious illness, if you are pregnant, or if you are a lactating mother.

By the way, fasting specifically helps cure addictions. Why? Because addictions leave incredible amounts of toxic buildup in the body. Gabriel Cousins, MD and dietary counselor, in his column in the September 1989 issue of *New Frontier Magazine*, said fasting is "excellent for helping addictions to food, cigarettes, and other drugs. When toxins are removed (by fasting), the cell memory of that to which one was addicted is changed. That is why the body tends to resist junk, polluted or artificial food and drugs after a fast."

Before choosing to fast, get more details. Learn as much as you can. Talk to a holistic dietary counselor or read more about it. One book that can help is Annemarie Colbin's *Food and Healing*.

INTESTINAL CLEANSING

If you have been a heavy drinker for many years, chances are you have some kind of bowel trouble. You may have irritable bowel syndrome, colitis, Crohn's disease, or chronic constipation.

The best ongoing treatment for these conditions is a good diet (as outlined in Chapter 6). But you may also benefit from colonic cleansing.

For starters, colonic cleansing solves one very serious problem: It removes built-up fecal matter that has lodged in the intestines over the course of years. Some people have up to five pounds of accumulated waste stuck to the lining of their intestines. Researchers associate the greatest fecal accumulations with diets high in fat, especially animal fat (meat, eggs, milk, butter, cheese, yogurt). Needless to say, this backlog of bodily waste impedes the normal functioning of the intestines and causes disease.

A colonic or enema can remove this buildup and give you a fresh start. No doubt you'll view this as good news. But keep in mind colonics or enemas should not be done too often.

Use a colonic maybe once a year or once every few years and consider it only if you have been eating poorly. An enema may be used occasionally to help with constipation. But if it is used too often, you can become dependent on it as easily as you can become dependent on laxatives.

If you choose this option, you may want to do it yourself. Or you may want to have it administered professionally. You can find many health resorts and holistic healing centers offering this service. Just check around.

HERBAL REMEDIES

Many plants and herbs have the power to heal. Ever since the dawn of civilization, these have been studied and classified. Indeed, for thousands of years these natural cures were the only medicines known.

Now, in the modern day, you can find herbal remedies for nearly any kind of complaint. Entire books have been devoted to the subject; you should use one of these books as a guide. (For instance, try *The Way of Herbs* by Michael Tierra, CA, ND, New York: Washington Square Press, 1980.) In addition, it may help you a great deal to get advice from a naturopathic doctor or other holistic health professional.

Meanwhile, to give you an idea, here are two lists of herbal health remedies: one for stress reduction, one to promote general physical healing.

Stress reducers

chamomile: relaxant, reduces anxiety, induces sleep

lady's slipper: reduces anxiety, lifts mood, helps cure depression

passionflower: sedative, induces sleep

St. John's wort: reduces anxiety, tension, and fatigue

skullcap: sedative, lifts depression, revitalizes nervous system

valerian: sedative, reduces tension

vervain: sedative, relieves depression and sadness

wood betony: relaxant, sedative, eases nervousness, relieves headaches due to nervousness

Internal healers

chaparral: antiseptic, antibiotic, stimulates the immune system

echinacea: antibiotic, good for acute infections, regulates white blood cell count

garlic: antibiotic, increases the body's resistance to infection

ginseng: strengthens the immune system, increases resistance to stress, builds stamina, renews sexual vitality

goldenseal: fights bacteria, helps cure infections, especially of throat and chest

marigold: stimulates white blood cell and interferon production

pau d'arco: anti-yeast, anti-fungal agent

peppermint: good for stomach ache, stimulates internal cleansing and strengthens the body

thyme: stimulates internal cleansing and strengthens the body

One caution: These herbs are very powerful. A little, once in a while, may be good for you, but too much can harm you. Use only as needed, until you experience the healing benefits, and then stop. Herbs can be taken with water or made into a mild tea and sipped.

AROMATHERAPY

For thousands of years, scents and fragrances have been used for healing and mood-changing purposes. Consider the atmosphere created by incense burning at a spiritual service, or the power of various perfumes and body lotions to stimulate sexual desire. Consider a fragrant potpourri that blithely lifts your mood, or the scent of a certain bath oil that totally relaxes you.

Aromatherapy is a form of herbal healing. You use various plants and herbs that impart active ingredients in their scent or aroma. By simply smelling or inhaling the active ingredients, you experience a physical change inside.

You can find aroma cures for many kinds of ailments. Here are a few that are recommended to alleviate depression and nervousness:

almond oil: relaxant, reduces nervousness

chamomile: mood lifter and relaxant

lavender: relaxant

lemon oil: mood lifter, reduces depression

melissa: relaxant

narcissus: relaxant

peppermint: mood lifter, reduces depression

pine oil: mood lifter

rose: mood lifter, calmative, reduces depression

sandalwood: relaxant

spearmint: mood lifter

ylang-ylang: relaxant

For best results, use the pure essential oils from these natural products. The oils can be simply smelled from the bottle, misted into the air, added to a hot bath, or gently massaged into your skin.

For more information on fragrances and many useful ideas, see *The Handbook of Aromatherapy* by Marcel Lavabre, or *The Art of Aromatherapy* by Robert B. Tisserand.

HOMEOPATHY

A complete health care system, homeopathy uses plant, mineral, and animal substances to stimulate healing. You can use this system not only to cure common ailments but to improve your general long-term health and well-being.

You won't find a specific cure for alcoholism. But you can use homeopathy to heal many of the ailments caused by alcoholism.

For additional information, see *Everybody's Guide to Homeopathic Medicine* by Dana Ullman, MPH. Or go to a homeopathic professional for specific remedies and advice.

CHIROPRACTIC

What comes to your mind when you think of chiropractic? Back problems, right? Well, chiropractic isn't just for back problems.

As you probably know, the spinal cord carries the main energy flow inside your body. By aligning spinal vertebrae, chiropractors enhance this energy flow, increasing "communication" through the spinal cord and all the peripheral nerves. This process in turn reduces stress and promotes inner healing, as the nerve networks and pathways are unblocked and resensitized.

Chiropractic offers one of the best methods of regaining health for the alcoholic whose nerves have been numbed by years of drinking.

Check for a chiropractor or chiropractic clinic near you.

A CHEMICAL DETERRENT TO DRINKING

If alcohol made you sick every time you drank it, you would probably not have become a drinker. You can actually make this happen. There is a drug that will not reduce your desire to drink, but will make you sick if you do. You've probably heard of it. It's disulfiram, marketed as Antabuse.

Some alcoholics find Antabuse helpful when they quit drinking. They need to feel there is one really powerful reason not to drink. Antabuse gives them this reason. If they take so much as a couple of sips, they'll get sick, perhaps even violently ill (vomiting, convulsing). So, in a practical way, Antabuse helps you gain control.

The main drawback? You must add a foreign chemical to your body. In the long run this may detract from your health.

Nevertheless, Antabuse may be for you. It may give you that extra boost, that extra feeling of self-control you need. Perhaps you can quit it after a year or two when you feel stronger.

If you want to start on Antabuse, go to a medical doctor. You need to take it under supervision—and you need a prescription.

ALTERNATIVE APPROACHES
TO QUITTING DRINKING

You already know about AA, which has dominated formal addiction treatment since the 1950s. Of course, most people who have quit serious alcoholic drinking have done so informally, without the ongoing use of any treatment program. As evidence of this, the book *The Day America Told the Truth* by researchers James Patterson and Peter Kim reveals that currently in the United States there are 19 million alcoholics in recovery and another 11 million alcoholics still drinking. From AA's own numbers, we know that AA has fewer than 1 million active members in the United States. That means approximately 95% of the alcoholics in recovery choose not to use AA. It also means that 29 million Americans might possibly be interested in some group program other than AA.

In this book, you have one of the new alternatives to the AA program. But many other programs are also available to you. Some of these are programs that offer a national network of groups which, like AA, meet in a regular place on a regular basis. And some of these are programs that individuals can use on their own.

Four Group Programs

You can call or write to any of these for more information or to find a meeting near you:

Women for Sobriety (WFS)
PO Box 618
Quakertown, PA 18951
215-536-8026
800-333-1606

- Founder: Jean Kirkpatrick, Ph.D.
- Started: 1975
- Number of members active in groups in U.S.: 5,000
- Number of groups in U.S.: 250
- Number of groups outside U.S.: 15
- Growth: This program has enjoyed a steady although gradual growth since its inception.
- Background: When Jean Kirkpatrick had quit her alcoholic drinking, she found that AA did not work for her. One reason: In mixed groups such as AA, men tend to dominate the discussion, which often leaves women feeling intimidated or frustrated. Yet what women need most in recovery is to build self-esteem.
- So WFS offers 13 Statements of Acceptance. In contrast to AA's 12 Steps, these are nonreligious thoughts to help members become more self-reliant in everyday life and to achieve a lasting and successful recovery.
- As part of its program, WFS offers recommendations to help with physical healing, including a dietary plan and guidelines for exercise. That means, among all the group programs including AA, WFS stands out as the only one to incorporate a whole-person approach.
- Books by Jean Kirkpatrick, Ph.D., about the program:
  Goodbye Hangovers, Hello Life: Self-Help for Women. New York: Atheneum, 1986.
  Turnabout: New Help for the Woman Alcoholic. New York: Bantam, 1990.

Men for Sobriety (MFS)
(address same as above)
Founder: Jean Kirkpatrick, Ph.D.

- Started: 1990
- Number of members active in groups: 100
- Number of groups: 10
- Growth: Very slow, gradual growth.
- Background: The WFS program works for men too. For instance, men find the 13 Statements of Acceptance to be strong esteem-boosters and, like women, can use them as helpful building blocks to a successful recovery.

Secular Organizations for Sobriety (SOS)
Also known as Save Our Selves
PO Box 5
Buffalo, NY 14215-0005
716-834-2922

- Founder: James Christopher
- Started: 1986
- Number of members active in groups in U.S.: 20,000
- Number of groups in U.S.: 1,200
- Number of members outside U.S. (SOS, in alliance with secular recovery groups in Europe): 80,000
- Number of groups outside U.S.: 4,000
- Growth: This popular program has grown steadily since its inception. It had a major growth spurt in foreign membership (in the early 1990s) through an alliance with secular recovery groups in Europe.
- Background: When Jim Christopher quit his own alcoholic drinking, he tried AA, only to find that it did not work for him. The main problem: the religiosity of the AA program. So he started SOS as a secular alternative.
- Instead of 12 Steps, SOS offers six Suggested Guidelines for Sobriety. These are powerful

ideas designed to help you take control of your life.

- Two keys to SOS: (1) Every day, you acknowledge that sobriety is your "Number 1" priority. This is called your Sobriety Priority. (2) You keep your own personal Journal of Recovery, a specifically designed workbook covering 52 weeks of the year. In SOS as well as various other programs, the journal technique has proven an extremely successful adjunct to recovery.
- Books by James Christopher:
  Unhooked: Staying Sober and Drug-Free. Buffalo: Prometheus Books, 1989.
  SOS Sobriety: The Proven Alternative to 12-Step Programs. Buffalo: Prometheus Books, 1992.

Rational Recovery (RR)
Box 800
Lotus, CA 95651
916-621-4374

- Founder: Jack Trimpey, LCSW
- Started: 1986
- Number of members active in groups in U.S.: 6,000
- Number of groups in U.S.: 600
- Number of groups outside U.S.: 50
- Growth: Very slow growth from 1986 to 1989. Since then, this program has grown more rapidly than any other group program in the country, including AA.
- Background: When Jack Trimpey tried to quit his own alcoholic drinking, AA did not work for him. He felt the moralizing of AA, the required religiosity, and the idea of powerlessness were

not helpful to most people and in fact could be detrimental to someone trying to make a constructive change. That's why he developed RR—to provide a "rational alternative."

- Based on the rational-emotive therapy (RET) developed by Dr. Albert Ellis, RR teaches its members to identify the addictive voice within, that inner voice that keeps urging you to drink, and to fight it. That's the irrational side of you, referred to as "the beast." RR gives you numerous methods to help you fight the beast and 14 Rational Ideas that you can use as guidelines to successful recovery.
- RR has another goal: to teach its members enough about RET so that they will be able to leave RR within a year to a year and a half and remain sober. In other words, RR does not foster any kind of dependency, including dependency on regular meetings. So far, RR has "graduated" many from its program (approximately 10,000 from 1986 to 1993); these graduates are always welcome to return to meetings whenever they feel a need.
- A recent study, reported in the *American Journal of Drug & Alcohol Abuse*, showed a six-month success rate for RR at 58%.
- See *The Small Book: A Revolutionary Alternative for Overcoming Alcohol and Drug Dependence* by Jack Trimpey. New York: Delacorte, 1992.

Individual Programs

Currently you can find at least 20 self-help programs that can be used as alternatives to AA. All have been described in books. Here are seven of the most notable:

Alcoholism, The Biochemical Connection: A Break-
through Seven-Week Self-Treatment Program by Joan
Mathews Larson, Ph.D. New York: Villard Books,
1992.

Mathews Larsen, the director of Health Recovery
Center in Minneapolis, uses this program with clients
at the center. A "biomedical regimen for recovery," it
offers a very strong component for physical healing.
Through diet and dietary supplements, you can heal
the body, eliminate addictive cravings, and even solve
problems with mood, such as depression. Proven success rate: 75%.

Help Yourself: A Revolutionary Alternative Recovery
Program by Dr. Joel C. Robertson. Nashville: Thomas
Nelson, 1992.

Dr. Robertson, director of the Robertson Institute,
Ltd., in Michigan, specializes in neuropharmacology
(brain chemistry technology). His book serves as an
in-depth workbook which will help you at all levels:
physical, emotional, mental, and spiritual. After you
determine your personal nature, you choose techniques to meet your specific needs.

A Million Dollars for Your Hangover by Maxie
Maultsby, Jr., MD. Lexington, KY: Rational Self-Help
Books, 1978.

Maultsby is currently the chairman of the department of psychiatry at Howard University Hospital in
Washington, DC. He is the creator of Rational Behavior Therapy (RBT) and the emotional self-help method
called Rational Self-Counseling. He also formulated
the new Self-Help Alcoholic Treatment Method.
Using RBT, you view alcoholism as a learned way of
coping. You unlearn your addiction by making a conscious choice not to drink and by learning new ways
to cope with life. (*A Million Dollars for Your Hang-*

over was one of his original books. Many newer books by Maultsby are also available. For information, write: International Association for Clear Thinking, 3939 W. Spencer Street, Appleton, WI 54914.)

Rational Madness: The Paradox of Addiction by Ray Hoskins. Blue Ridge Summit, PA: Tab Books, 1989.

This book presents an extremely enlightening view of addictive behavior. When you peel away one layer of addiction (such as alcohol or drug addiction), you find other layers of addiction (for instance, food addictions, various mental compulsions, as well as "behavior addictions," such as the addiction to work, gambling, sex, and relationships). The book offers techniques, primarily psychological and spiritual, to help you work through these layers of addiction and become free.

The Recovery Book by Al J. Mooney, MD, Arlene Eisenberg, and Howard Eisenberg. New York: Workman, 1992.

This giant 600-page guide looks at all aspects of recovery. In it, AA gets mentioned often as a recovery technique, but the book answers hundreds of questions about recovery in non-AA terms. You'll find that this book serves very much as an encyclopedia, covering the entire recovery field with useful information and state-of-the-art advice.

Recovery from Addiction by John Finnegan and Daphne Gray. Berkeley, CA: Celestial Arts, 1990.

The authors urge a whole-person approach to recovery and give suggestions to guide the reader. This book presents a strong dietary plan, along with some recipes for you to try. It also includes nutritional and herbal therapy to help treat various medical problems that you encounter in recovery.

The Truth About Addiction and Recovery: The Life-Process Program for Outgrowing Destructive Habits by Stanton Peele, Ph.D., and Archie Brodsky with Mary Arnold. New York: Simon & Schuster, 1991.

With the Life Process Program, you assess the impact of addiction(s) on your life. Then you take a look at what's really important to you. By doing this, you can answer the question "Do I need to make a change?" If the answer is yes, the book gives you a complete set of guidelines to help you change behavior, including "life skills" training. This book offers a lifestyle-change approach to quitting addictions, a type of approach that has proven extremely effective in numerous studies.

COUNSELING/PSYCHOTHERAPY

When you're feeling down or upset, what's more helpful than a sympathetic ear? A good listener can comfort you, make you feel strong, and give you a sense that someone is on your side. What's more, a good therapy session can help you find solutions to your problems.

Counseling can help you with many kinds of problems. A CAC (certified alcoholism counselor) can help you specifically with quitting drinking. Most counselors or psychotherapists can help you improve your emotional condition in general . . . or help you specifically to reduce anxiety, relieve depression, enrich your relationships with others, and improve your attitude toward yourself.

Today, most health insurance policies cover counseling and psychotherapy. More and more people have been trying it and getting good results. If you give it a try, you may find it can be very beneficial for you as well.

How do you find the right counselor? Be prepared to shop around. You want a counselor you feel compatible with, one you can talk to comfortably, and so on. Keep looking until you find one who definitely helps you.

GROUP THERAPY

How would you feel if you could share your feelings in a group and be accepted for what you are? Pretty good, right? That's because a group has a certain self-affirming influence on everyone in it.

Like psychotherapy, group therapy can help you with specific behaviors. For instance, you can find groups to help you with stress reduction, groups for people who have lost a loved one, groups for people with a serious disease such as cancer, and so on.

If the 12 Steps work for you, you can find an "Anonymous" group for almost anything: Alcoholics Anonymous, Narcotics Anonymous, Codependents Anonymous, Adult Children of Alcoholics (Anonymous), Gamblers Anonymous, Overeaters Anonymous, Sex Addicts Anonymous, Child Abusers Anonymous, and more. Also, in the section "Alternative Approaches to Quitting Drinking" in this chapter, you learned about some alternative groups: Women for Sobriety, Rational Recovery, and Secular Organizations for Sobriety. Here's another group that you could try: the International Association for Clear Thinking (I'ACT). I'ACT groups offer self-counseling methods to help you increase your personal happiness. You can find many groups meeting in different cities in the United States. (For information, contact I'ACT, 3939 W. Spencer Street, Appleton, WI 54914, phone 414-739-8311.) Otherwise, to find different types of psychotherapy groups, check with local mental health clinics and psychotherapists in private practice.

If given a chance, the right group can open you to parts of yourself that you haven't seen before. The right group can help you feel safe around others. Furthermore, the right group can help you solve problems about yourself that will improve your overall approach to life. When you think about it, it might be worth your time to find some kind of group therapy that's just right for you.

When seeking a group, follow the same rules for finding a counselor or therapist. Shop around for a group that focuses specifically on your problems, one in which you feel comfortable, one that will help you grow.

LIGHT THERAPY

The sun's energy is what makes life on earth possible. Light from the sun spurs important biochemical processes: photosynthesis in plants, for instance, and the production of vitamin D in humans.

Sunlight has been linked to human emotions. For instance a normal amount of natural sunlight, on a regular basis, promotes happiness. The less sunlight people get, the more depressed they become. Without natural full-spectrum lighting, work performance declines, erratic behavior and nervousness increase, and the likelihood of disease is greater (everything from routine headaches to life-threatening cancers).

What kind of light causes problems? Any kind

that deviates too much from the natural full-spectrum light given off by the sun. For instance, almost any kind of indoor (artificial) lighting causes problems. This includes conventional electric light bulbs and almost all fluorescent lighting.

More than a hundred studies show that people do better at almost any task—and report feeling better—under full-spectrum lighting as opposed to any other form of lighting. Most artificial lighting concentrates in only one or two bands of the spectrum. Full-spectrum lighting blends all bands of the spectrum.

Of course, sunlight is the best (and original) source of full-spectrum lighting. Plan to expose yourself to some sunlight every day—not too much, maybe about a half-hour a day. You don't even have to sit directly in the sun—indirect sunlight works fine. That means you can sit in the shade of a porch or under a tree and still gain the benefits. Get outside even when it's cold. You might be bundled up, but the sun still dances in your eyes. A daily dose of sunlight does wonders for your disposition. Try it; you'll see.

Aside from enjoying natural sunlight, make sure to change your indoor lighting. For full-spectrum lighting, try Ott-Lites from Lumax Industries, PO Box 991, Altoona, PA 16603. Send for a catalog. Or buy Chromolux full-spectrum light bulbs from Lumiram Electric Corporation. You can find them in stores that carry health products.

EXPRESSIVE ARTS THERAPY

Alcohol addiction stifles creativity. Studies show that creativity—the ability for creative thought—diminishes in heavy drinkers. But when you quit drinking, your creativity will gradually return. So, as you recover, you need to channel your new-found creativity. It's there, waiting to be tapped. You can use it to help you make money or simply to enjoy yourself.

Some addiction-recovery centers have now added "artistic expression" as a vital part of treatment. The reason: It has been proven successful in recovery. You can participate in a program at one of these centers, take various classes in your local community, or work with your creativity on your own.

First of all, decide how you want to channel your creative energy. What form of artistic expression do you like? Drawing, painting, sculpting, pottery, crafts, photography, music, writing (including journal writing), dance, acting? Each one gives you an outlet and will help you feel more fulfilled. Each one offers the opportunity to express something deep inside you.

Choose one or more. Then get into it. Let your creativity flow. Don't hold back. Show your emotions through your form of artistry. Enjoy the freedom of creative expression.

HUG A FRIEND

Your sense of touch has a profound effect on your emotional life. Ever notice how a friendly touch can warm you? Touch someone and see. The feel of another person can be calming and reassuring. A simple hug reduces stress.

After working with alcoholics and other addicts for over 50 years, Dr. Eugene Scheimann has come to believe that people become addicted to alcohol or drugs as a substitute for touch. Addiction happens when we feel "out of touch," when we feel we cannot give or get the physical affection we need.

What can we do? Try:

- trading massages with a friend or loved one.
- holding hands with your lover in the movies or on a walk.
- hugging a friend.
- patting your buddy on the back.
- kissing and hugging your loved ones . . . whenever and as often as you can.

This is therapeutic touch at its best. It's intimate. It's personal. It has the power of love and friendship behind it. Of course, you can go for a professional massage or some other kind of hands-on therapy and it will help too.

But get your sense of touch out of the closet. Act as if every day is National Hug a Friend Day. Occasionally, for a change, pretend it's National Hug a Enemy Whether You Like It or Not Day. Touch as many lives as you can.

RELIGION

There are more than 100 different religions in this world. Each has its own beauty. Each one supports a certain lifestyle and offers its own unique wisdom to humankind.

Any of these religions could be right for you. Which one do you like? For starters, here's a list of major religions:

Buddhism	Hinduism
Christianity	Islam

Jainism	Sufism
Judaism	Taoism
Shinto	Zen
Sikhism	Zoroastrianism

Plus you can add many major religions of the ancient world, such as the early pantheistic religions of Greece, Rome, Egypt, and Mesopotamia.

And there are the dozens upon dozens of colorful, yet deeply rich, tribal religions found all over North and South America, Asia, Australia, Africa, and on every major island.

You may want to check out some of these other religions, especially if you question your present religion. You may find one that better suits your temperament and lifestyle. But even if you don't, the search in itself can be rewarding.

Of course, you may want to return to your original faith, the religion of your youth. Many people who quit their alcohol addiction become totally reabsorbed in their original faith. The reason: They find a sense of personal renewal. When asked what's different the second time around, many report that they finally found themselves "letting go." What do they mean? Letting go of their problems, letting go of their struggle, giving in to faith. In AA, there's an expression that seems apt here, "Let go and let God."

So how do you feel about religion? Is it an experience you will want to nurture?

The right religion can help you find peace and love, joy and inner strength. Indeed, the experience can be truly beautiful. But there's one more thing. You will discover that religion, by launching you into the spiritual realm, will help set you free.

SPIRITUAL HEALING

You don't necessarily need religion to help you feel free. Many techniques designed to improve your spiritual growth can do it too.

Alcohol stifles spiritual growth. Most heavy drinkers remain spiritually lost their entire drinking careers. It doesn't matter how old you are—when you start drinking heavily, you stop growing spiritually. When you quit the alcohol, spiritual growth begins again.

So be prepared for the change. Plan to pursue some form of spiritual growth soon after you quit drinking. Be prepared ahead of time to make some new spiritual connection.

Then, as you make the change, watch what happens. You begin to view the world through different eyes. A fundamental shift in attitude occurs. Deep inside, you experience a new verve for life. You gain a fresh view of the world and develop a revitalized commitment to life.

How will you make this change? You can get involved in religion (see preceding section), try a 12-step program, or use any of the spiritual techniques.

Meditation & Meditative Techniques

Yogic meditation. Usually performed in a seated, cross-legged posture. You clear the mind to focus on one thing, such as your breath, a sound (mantra), an image (yantra), or on nothingness.

Zazen, Zen meditation. Often done in a kneeling position. You may focus on a koan (an illogical thought intended to break through the logical mind, such as "What is the sound of one hand clapping?"). Or you may focus on dropping the mind, by letting go of each thought as it arises.

Zen archery. You don't shoot the arrow . . . the arrow shoots itself. You are merely a medium through which it occurs.

Sufi whirling. Method of dancing by spinning like a top. Induces a deep meditative state.

Yoga sutras. Over a hundred separate techniques, little meditative tricks, to help you gain a glimpse of ultimate reality. See *The Book of Secrets*, five volumes, by Bhagwan Shree Rajneesh, or *The Yoga Sutras of Patanjali* by M. N. Dvivedi.

Rajneesh meditations. Incorporating the best from East and West, Rajneesh developed about 20 powerful meditations designed to awaken your spiritual self. Each of these meditations takes about an hour to do, usually in three to five parts, alternating Western "active" exercise with Eastern "passive" meditation postures. The result: exceptional relaxation . . . euphoria . . . peace, contentment . . . feelings of at-one-ment. See *The Orange Book* by Bhagwan Shree Rajneesh.

Prayer

Often done kneeling. Prayers help you to connect with a higher power by directing your thoughts to that power. You may offer thanks, supplication, or devotion. You may request forgiveness or ask for help. Most moments of prayer are solemn, accompanied by a meditative state of mind.

Many Paths of Yoga

You may choose many techniques but have only one path. The path you choose relates to your general outlook, a consistent pattern of behavior that works well for you. As you change, your path may change. Some examples of paths:

Hatha yoga. You work with, and gain mastery over, breath, health, and the physical body.

Bhakti. You gain mastery over love and devotion, opening yourself to a higher consciousness. (For those who live more in the heart.)

Jnana yoga. You use your power of intellect to learn possibilities, to sort through alternatives and to gain knowledge. Sometimes it takes a great deal of knowledge to realize how useless knowledge really is. (For those who live more in the mind.)

Karma yoga. You become at one with your work or principal activity. You reach contentment through creating and producing various positive changes in the world.

Tantra. A method of feeling at one with whatever you happen to be doing at any given moment. You totally immerse yourself in the details of each and every moment. You achieve ecstasy by living each moment now.

Rebirthing

One of the newest methods of spiritual healing involves using visualization and special breathing techniques to relive the moment of your birth. This time around, however, you undo all the fear and trauma accompanying your original birth. After a successful rebirthing you feel as if you have been born again, only with a greater love and acceptance than before. Check local holistic health centers or new age directories for certified rebirthing practitioners in your area.

The Art of Surrender

When you give your self up, you can live anew. Think of your self for a moment . . . think of everything you imagine your self to be. Now give it up. Throw this self away. It means nothing. Without this self demanding things, you have nothing to fight for, nothing to fear. As a result, you accept life and feel at one with it.

Hence a new different self, a more accepting self, begins to emerge. But keep in mind, if this self becomes selfish and demanding, if it wants to take over your life and the lives of others, drop it. Even though this new self might be fighting for a "good cause," a better cause than your former self, drop it. Surrender it too. Every time a self becomes fixated on something and begins to claim too much, move on. Leave it. That way, you'll continue to grow.

CHARITY/ALTRUISM

Do a good deed. Help somebody out, really help somebody, and you begin to feel warm inside. Your heart's aglow. You settle into a moment or two of peaceful contentment.

Try it. You don't just create these feelings in your mind. They're real. An actual change takes place inside. But not only do you feel better emotionally, you become stronger physically. In a study of 2,700 people, over a ten-year period, researchers found that doing regular volunteer work, more than any other activity, increased life expectancy.

But that's not all. Offering a helping hand may actually help to heal you. In his best-selling book *Love, Medicine and Miracles*, Dr. Bernie Siegel reports that doing something for someone else boosts immune-system activity. Indeed, compared to all options, it may be one of the best immune-system boosters available.

It all comes down to one simple act: giving. Give some of your time, give some of your energy, give some of the fruits of your labor to help another. It's bound to make you smile.

The Boy Scouts have a good slogan, "Do a good turn daily." You may want to make it your slogan too. Meanwhile, keep in mind another popular slogan, "Helping you helps me."

GROWING IN LOVE

Love is the ultimate opening of the heart. Love is relationships . . . giving . . . bhakti yoga . . . family togetherness. God is love.

Love brings spiritual awakening. And any spiritual awakening brings love.

When you open in love, you begin to bloom. You offer your self completely, without reservation. In truth, the self dissolves . . . melts into the object of your affection. This is a love of total giving. This love frees you from your psychic chains.

A selfish love won't do. A possessive love won't

do. These are neurotic forms of love—destructive, draining, incomplete.

The love of giving, the love that's pure of heart, can be for one other. It can be for God. It can be your love for all others, all living things, the entire universe.

It is an opening of the heart, a giving of the self, a maturing. It releases the true self, an uncluttered self, a selfless self, the self of the soul. Some brilliance from deep within comes shining through.

Allow yourself love. Let go into it. Free yourself within it. Open yourself to all the world.

To get a better feel for it, read *Love* by Leo Buscaglia; *Loving Relationships* by Sondra Ray; and *Love Is Letting Go of Fear* by Gerald Jampolsky.

Meanwhile, here's one parting thought on the subject of love:

> *Love and the self are one and the discovery of either is the realization of both.*
>
> —*from* Love *by Leo Buscaglia*

Worksheet #7

Which Techniques Will You Do?

Instructions: Study the following groups. Then choose at least one technique from each group.

Select only techniques that you will do. *Then do them.* Plan to be doing all six techniques by the end of your second month away from alcohol. (Do more than six techniques, if you want, by choosing any additional techniques you would like to do.)

Group 1
- ☐ acupuncture/CES
- ☐ massage
- ☐ biofeedback
- ☐ bodywork/body movement
- ☐ hypnosis

Group 2
- ☐ autogenic training/self-hypnosis
- ☐ visualization
- ☐ affirmations
- ☐ subliminal suggestion

Group 3
- ☐ a clinic or a live-in program
- ☐ solitude and self-reflection
- ☐ healing with laughter
- ☐ turn off the TV

Group 4
- ☐ fasting
- ☐ intestinal cleansing
- ☐ herbal remedies
- ☐ aromatherapy
- ☐ homeopathy
- ☐ chiropractic
- ☐ a chemical deterrent to drinking
- ☐ alternative approaches to quitting drinking
- ☐ counseling/psychotherapy
- ☐ group therapy

Group 5
- ☐ light therapy
- ☐ expressive art therapy
- ☐ hug a friend

Group 6
- ☐ religion
- ☐ spiritual healing
- ☐ charity/altruism
- ☐ growing in love

PART THREE

Quitting and Making It Work for You

CHAPTER 9

Okay—Pick a Day

Nothing is so perfectly amusing as a total change of ideas.

—*Laurence Sterne*

N ow it's time to take action. It's time to quit drinking and put everything you've learned so far to use.

Ever been in jail? The alcohol addiction is like being in jail. You're stuck . . . locked in. You've lost your freedom. But there's an interesting twist. *You* have the key—the key to your own jail cell! All you have to do is let yourself out. By quitting drinking, you let yourself out.

By now you're probably looking forward to it. Physically, you need the change. Emotionally, you're ready for it.

Plus you've got all the information you need to be successful. If you quit drinking now and do all the things you have learned so far, you won't even think about alcohol. If you can do just half the things you've learned, that's still enough to guarantee your success.

Here's what you'll do in this chapter:

- Draw up a Master Plan—all the things you will do to help you when you quit.

- Make a promise to quit drinking.
- Sign a contract to quit.
- Pick a day and quit drinking on that day.

By the end of this chapter you will free yourself from alcohol and start a brand-new life.

USE EVERYTHING YOU'VE LEARNED SO FAR

A little knowledge may be a dangerous thing, but the right amount can help you move mountains. Right now you have enough knowledge to quit drinking and begin moving mountains. By way of a simple review, Worksheet #8 shows the most important changes you need to make. Use it to jog your memory.

Worksheet #8

Your Master Plan

Instructions: Review the key elements in your program for quitting. Check each one you have begun. Begin doing anything you haven't yet started.

☐ Stop denying the problems caused by alcohol (Chapter 2, Worksheet #1).

☐ Look at the problems again. Remember how much you'd like to avoid these problems (Chapter 3, Worksheet #3).

☐ Your reasons for quitting. Carry with you a written list of your most important reasons (Chapter 3, Worksheet #4).

☐ Follow your decision about AA (Chapter 4, Worksheet #5).

- ☐ Remember your alternatives to drinking. Start doing them the day you quit (Chapter 5, Checklist #2).
- ☐ Change your diet (Chapter 6, Practice #4).
- ☐ Start your exercise program (Chapter 7, Practice #5).
- ☐ Use your relaxation techniques (Chapter 7, Checklist #3).
- ☐ Become more assertive (Chapter 7, Practice #6).
- ☐ Reduce stress (Chapter 7, Checklist #4).
- ☐ Talk with a friend (Chapter 7, Practice #7).
- ☐ Start additional techniques to renew yourself (Chapter 8, Worksheet #7).

PROMISE SOMEONE

The next important step is to promise someone close to you that you will quit drinking. Do it in writing.

Choose someone who is very close to you—a family member, a lover, or a friend—preferably someone who has urged you to quit drinking, someone who wants you to get better. Write this person a letter promising that you will quit drinking. (Note: If you can't think of anyone, do this exercise by making a promise to yourself.)

Tell that person your most important reason for quitting. Say that you will quit drinking soon and promise that you will stay away from alcohol after you quit. Explain that you want to begin enjoying your life and not continue to ruin it. Affirm that you want to gain all the benefits of not drinking.

Write down all of this and make a copy of it. Give the original to your friend, lover, or family member. Put the copy under your pillow.

MAKE A CONTRACT

Here's a quick and simple way to put more power into your commitment: Promise yourself that you will do it. Make a vow to yourself that you will stick to it. Make it your solemn oath. Then write it in a contract.

This last idea is perhaps the most important. When you write your vow into a contract and sign it, it becomes formal. It becomes a solid plan. It gives you something to live up to.

Worksheet #9

Contract to Quit Drinking

Instructions: You may use the following contract as is, or rewrite it in your own words. If you want to rewrite it, do that now. When you pick your date to quit, put that in your contract and sign it. In addition, you may choose someone close to you to witness your contract. This can be very helpful, but make sure to choose someone who will offer you encouragement.

It's a good idea to make a copy of your contract and hang it on your wall where you will see it every morning.

Contract

I, _____ (name) promise to stop drinking on _____ (date). I promise to follow my Master Plan to ensure my success.

I will use the techniques that I've learned in *How to Quit Drinking Without AA* to review my progress regularly and to strengthen my commitment each day.

I will treat this contract as a solemn oath, my vow, my personal commitment to myself.

Date: _____ Signed: _____

Witness (optional): _____

Some optional lines you can add to your contract:
- I will not drink just for today.
- I will not drink for this very minute.
- I promise that if my heart is beating, I will not drink.

PICK A DAY AND QUIT

Now you can get down to business. It's time. If you quit drinking today and use everything you've learned so far, you will succeed.

Admittedly, it won't be easy at first. You will have to make a lot of changes all at once. But you can do it. Remember: Millions of people have quit drinking successfully—and most of them had less practical information than you have.

Say When

The day you quit can be of key importance. By choosing your own day, you stay in control. You can take a little time to plan for it. You can get in the right frame of mind.

People who don't plan tend to quit after a horrible drunk—a bout of drinking that shows beyond a doubt how serious their problems really are. Maybe they nearly got themselves killed. Maybe they hurt someone badly. Or woke up in jail. Or had to be hospitalized.

If any of these happens—just once—it's too much. Don't wait for it to happen to you. It's like flirting with death. It may kill you.

You don't have to wait for an alcohol-induced tragedy to jar you awake. You already know all the problems caused by excessive drinking. You know how serious these problems are. Why wait for them to get worse? Look at it this way: If you knew you had cancer and you knew the cure, would you wait for the cancer to spread more before starting the cure?

So . . . when should you quit? As soon as possible. You're ready. You're as ready as you'll ever be. Your body needs a break and there's no better time than now to get your life in order.

If you need inpatient care for detox, plan for it. Tell people and arrange for your responsibilities to be taken care of. Take vacation or sick leave from work, and enter a detox center.

Even if you don't go for inpatient care, take a couple of weeks off. You'll find things go easier if you drop your normal routine.

In addition, please keep this in mind: Quitting is serious business. If you approach it seriously, you'll be stronger, more committed to getting good results. For this reason, don't bet money. It can put undue pressure on you. And don't make any grand announcements. Don't go around telling *everyone* you're going to quit. This adds pressure too. When it's your time to quit, quit quietly.

Now ask yourself this question: What's the best time—in the near future—for me to quit drinking? Pick one day out of the next 30 days. Next week? Two weeks from now? The last weekend of the month? Make your date and stick to it.

Worksheet #10

Your Day

Instructions: Write the day and date you choose to quit drinking. You may drink the day before . . . but on this date you will not drink. Then every day thereafter, you will not drink.

What day of the week did you pick? _____
What is the date (month/day/year)? _____

Now put the date you will quit in your contract to quit . . . and sign it.

CHAPTER 10

Getting a Successful Start

"Toto, I have a feeling we're not in Kansas any-more."

—Dorothy, *in* The Wizard of Oz

If you were a rocket ship waiting to be launched, a group of experts would clear you. "All systems go," they would say, each in their turn, when asked whether you were ready for takeoff.

You can use this technique on yourself. When you quit drinking, immediately you need to clear yourself on three points. You need to know:

- how to cope with urges.
- how to keep the right distance between you and alcohol.
- what to say when offered a drink.

In the three sections of this chapter, you will check yourself on these important points.

COPING WITH URGES

It's going happen. Every so often you'll get the urge to take a drink. What will you do about it? How many ways do you know to help you cope with this urge?

How about 164? That's right. You know 164 ways to reduce, eliminate, or change the urge to drink. In Checklist #2 (Chapter 5), you learned 112 alternatives to drinking. In Checklist #4 (Chapter 7), you learned 22 surefire stress reducers. In Chapter 8, you studied 30 healing techniques.

Pick one. Do any of the healing techniques, any of the stress reducers, any of your alternatives to drinking, and you'll forget the desire to drink. Or use any of the following five ways to cope with urges:

1. *Outlast it.* An urge remains strong for only five to ten minutes. Simply wait it out.

2. *View it as a power play that you can win.* Don't let an urge take control. Fight it. Show that you're more powerful. Get mad at the urge if you need to. Argue with it. Get in control. Win.

3. *Cut out the sweets.* If you keep eating and drinking sugar foods, you'll keep craving alcohol. Break the sugar habit—you'll feel much better.

4. *Change your routine.* People often drink as part of a certain routine, such as watching TV or talking on the phone to friends. So break any routine that you associate with drinking. Instead of watching TV, read a book or go for a walk. Instead of talking on the phone to friends, go visit them.

5. *Use mind over matter.* You can actually talk

yourself out of an urge by looking at the facts. First remember how bad your life had gotten before quitting drinking. Compare that to the life you have now—and consider the benefits you've gained by not drinking. Or remember your worst drunk—think of the trouble you caused yourself or someone else. Think about how bad it really was. Then consider this: No matter how bad things get now, you can always make them worse by drinking. This viewpoint can help you make a powerful decision to stay away from alcohol.

Worksheet #11

---

169 Ways to Cope with Urges

Instructions: Review your favorite methods of coping. See:

- Checklist #2, Chapter 5
- Checklist #4, Chapter 7
- Worksheet #7, Chapter 8
- the five ways listed above, this section

Now pick your favorite 20 ways to cope with urges. Write each of these in your notebook or on a separate piece of paper. Review them often. Use when necessary.

HOW CLOSE CAN YOU GET TO ALCOHOL?

When you quit drinking, your relationship with alcohol changes immediately. For a moment, think of alcohol as a person. You were in love with this person. In fact, you had an intimate relationship. But this person treated you badly. Very badly. This person hurt you emotionally and abused you physically.

Now you have broken the relationship. You have escaped. You're free. So what happens next?

Perhaps your emotion turns from love to hate. Maybe you hate alcohol now. Maybe you prefer to avoid having alcohol anywhere near you.

Or maybe you can part as "friends." Maybe you and alcohol cannot get along in a close relationship— you know you can't touch each other—but maybe you can be in the same room together.

It's up to you to decide.

Now that you've quit drinking, what's your new relationship with alcohol? How close can you get to a bottle without being tempted to drink?

Practice #8

Avoiding Drinking Situations

Instructions: Consider each question carefully, then answer it. If you have any doubts, leave it blank. If you know you can handle a situation, check the box in front of the question.

☐ Can you hold an open bottle two inches from your nose without being tempted?

☐ Can you hold a drink in your hand without being tempted?

☐ Can you walk within three feet of a drink without being tempted?

☐ Can you keep beer in the refrigerator or alcohol in the liquor cabinet without being tempted?

☐ Can you go to a bar without being tempted?

☐ Can you go to a social event and watch people drink without being tempted?

☐ Can you go to a party where friends are drinking without being tempted?

☐ Can a family member or friend drink alcohol near you without tempting you?

☐ Can you go to a restaurant where drinks are served without being tempted?

☐ Can you walk or drive past a liquor store without wanting to go in?

How Close Can You Get?

If you think you'll have trouble with a situation, avoid it. Avoid it as best you can.

Make plans to avoid it. Make excuses to avoid it. If you can't avoid a certain social function, go—but leave early if you don't feel comfortable. Meanwhile, practice your reasons for not drinking (Checklist #5, later in this chapter), and be ready to tell them to anyone, at any time.

In addition, you can use the following contract whenever you feel a need:

Non-Drinking Contract for a Specific Situation

I promise not to drink during _____ (specific situation) on _____ (date). I will remain levelheaded in the situation. And no matter what happens, I will choose not to drink.

Signed: _____ Date: _____

And Remember: You Get Stronger and Stronger

When you first quit drinking, many situations will seem hard for you. You will often feel tempted to drink. But as time goes by, you'll feel tempted less and less. It doesn't take very long—especially when you work to improve your health. Soon you will find it easy to be around alcohol without being tempted at all.

Just give yourself the time and allow things to change.

FOR ANYONE WHO ASKS YOU . . .

What will you say when someone asks, "Do you want to have a drink?" You can bet your life that many people will ask you. Do you know what to tell them?

When you quit drinking, it helps to have a few ways to say, "No, thanks." It helps to have a few solid excuses for not drinking. You almost need to talk about alcohol in a whole new light. Instead of talking about how much you want it or need it, you need to talk about why you don't want it, why you don't need it, or why you can't have it.

Think about it. Do you know, for instance, what you will tell your friends? What will you say to a friend who urges you to have a drink? What will you tell your date tonight? What about your family—what will you tell them?

Try this: Say to yourself a few times, "I don't drink." Practice it. Say it silently. Now say it out loud a few times. After you quit drinking, repeat this phrase to yourself often. And be ready to repeat it to others whenever the issue arises. You'll probably use some of these variations:

No, thanks, I don't drink.

No, I quit drinking.

Thanks, but I don't drink anymore.

Oh, didn't you know? I don't drink.

When people ask, sometimes you'll give a reason for not drinking . . . sometimes you'll give an excuse.

A reason for not drinking tells why you don't drink at all. A reason may tell people why you've quit drinking and why you don't plan to drink again. Example: "No, thanks, I stopped drinking because it was causing too many health problems."

An excuse covers you for one night or for one drink at a time. Example: "No, thanks, I'd rather dance." If you don't want to get into any personal details with people, you can simply make excuses. You can make excuses from now until you die . . . and never take a drink.

By the way, with excuses you can make up anything. An excuse doesn't have to be true—just effective. Have fun with it. Blow people's minds. Laugh about it . . .

Checklist #5

Why I'm Not Drinking

Instructions: Review these *reasons* and *excuses* for not drinking. Select any that you would feel comfortable using and put a check next to them.

Now go back through the list and put a second check next to those you like the most. Write these on a separate piece of paper. These are your favorite reasons and excuses for not drinking. Practice them. Be ready to use them anytime, in any situation, whenever needed.

Reasons

☐ Alcohol nearly killed me.

☐ I had to quit to save my life.

☐ My liver got so bad I had to quit.

☐ I have already drunk enough in my life.

- [ ] I have already drunk as much in my life as ten normal people.
- [ ] I have already drunk enough in my life to kill a normal person.
- [ ] I nearly got fired from work. I had to quit drinking to save my job.
- [ ] I got very sick from alcohol and I need to heal myself.
- [ ] I had an awful scrape with the law and had to quit drinking to stay out of jail.
- [ ] Drinking was screwing me up totally . . . making me crazy. I had to quit.
- [ ] I was losing my mind with alcohol.
- [ ] I was having too many fights with my wife . . . my husband . . . my kids.
- [ ] I had to quit drinking because I was afraid I might hurt somebody.
- [ ] Things were really getting bad. I had to quit drinking to turn my life around.
- [ ] Drinking was robbing me of energy. I could hardly do anything.
- [ ] Alcohol was making me a nervous wreck. I had to quit.
- [ ] I quit drinking because I want to set a good example for my children. I really care about them.
- [ ] I quit drinking to regain my health.
- [ ] Drinking was blocking my thinking. I quit so I could think clearly again.
- [ ] I quit to gain control of my life.
- [ ] I needed to get free. I felt like alcohol was holding me in a cage.
- [ ] I needed to regain my creativity.
- [ ] I needed to avoid pancreatitis.
- [ ] I had to reduce my blood pressure.
- [ ] I was drinking so much it caused internal bleeding.
- [ ] I had to quit.
- [ ] I had severe hypoglycemia and had to quit.

☐ I had _____ (serious physical condition) and had to quit drinking to save myself.

_____

_____

_____

_____

Excuses

☐ No, thanks, I'm the designated driver tonight.

☐ No, thanks, I just had one. (Feel free to lie. Any excuse is okay, as long as it keeps you from drinking.)

☐ No, thanks, I'm fine.

☐ No, thanks, I'm half-drunk already. (Remember, you can make up any lie you want.)

☐ No, thanks, I'm out of my mind as it is.

☐ Things are bad enough. I'd only make them worse by drinking.

☐ My doctor said I can't drink.

☐ I'm taking Antabuse. I can't touch a drop.

☐ I'd rather dance.

☐ I can't drink. I have too much to do tomorrow.

☐ No, thanks, I have to get up early tomorrow.

☐ No, thanks, I was just leaving.

☐ No, thanks, I'm not drinking today.

☐ Not today . . . I need a day off from the stuff.

☐ No, thanks, I promised _____ that I wouldn't drink today.

☐ I promised myself I wouldn't drink today and I'm going to keep my promise.

☐ It's done me in. I couldn't handle another drop.

☐ My _____ (sickness, internal problem) has been acting up and I can't touch a drop today.

☐ No, just give me a club soda with lime please. And no ice. Thank you.

☐ No, I'm on the wagon today.

☐ Can't you tell? I've become a teetotaler . . . give me a cup of tea.

☐ Just for the hell of it, I'm not going to drink today.

☐ Maybe you expected me to say yes, but no, I don't want a drink. Thanks anyway.

☐ Not right now, thanks.

☐ I can't possibly have a drink right now, and I can't even begin to tell you why. Just give me a club soda instead, please.

☐ It seems to bother you that I'm not drinking. You keep asking me to have a drink. If it bothers you that much, I'd better be going. See you later.

☐ No, thanks, I don't drink.

_____

_____

_____

CHAPTER 11

Fifteen Common Problems and How to Solve Them

All things are difficult before they are easy.
—Thomas Fuller, MD

After quitting drinking, 15 common problems arise. Everybody experiences them. By knowing what to expect, you can be prepared.

Two kinds of problems occur: (1) those that alcohol caused and (2) those that alcohol concealed. The problems alcohol caused relate to physical health. As a general rule, the more alcohol consumed, the worse your health becomes. For these problems, you need to revitalize your body and give it time to heal.

The problems alcohol concealed relate to emotions. These are the emotional problems you never really faced, the real life problems alcohol helped you forget. When you quit drinking, they reappear.

Now it's time to face both kinds of problems. It's

time to stop hiding, time for you to confront your problems head-on—and resolve them without alcohol. The following descriptions tell you what to expect and give you some realistic ways to resolve each individual problem.

ANXIETY

Feel nervous? Tense? That's a normal reaction to quitting drinking. Alcohol had you sedated for a long time. When you take the alcohol away, your nervous system gets highly active.

What's worse, if you used alcohol to calm yourself whenever you felt tense, now instead, the tension comes through full force. How will you cope with it now that you can't take a drink?

First, remember diet. Cut out all sweets. Don't even use artificial or substitute sweeteners. And cut out caffeine. Second, get a lot of exercise. Exercise relieves tension. Third, use stress reduction techniques. Especially try yoga or other forms of bodywork/body movement. Other possibilities: acupuncture, massage, biofeedback, herbal remedies, and aromatherapy. All can help reduce anxiety.

DEPRESSION

Everyone experiences some sadness in life and seeks ways to cope with it. Heavy drinkers use alcohol to cope. Maybe you used alcohol to forget some of your sad memories.

When you stop drinking, you must face your sadness head-on. Now is your time to deal with it in a realistic manner.

What works? Exercise. A brisk walk or a highly active workout relieves depression. Yoga does the same and it increases your mental power as well. What else? Talk with a friend or counselor. Use visualization, affirmations, or self-hypnosis. Turn off the TV. Or try light therapy, expressive art therapy, and charity (doing something for others). In your diet, stay away from sweets.

ANGER

Heavy drinking is one of the main causes of anger. Now that you've quit drinking, you probably get less angry, although you may still have some problems with this intense emotion. Most likely, you'll find that anger has its emotional roots deep in your childhood. For this reason, counseling, psychotherapy, or group therapy may help.

Otherwise you can alter the biochemical triggers to your anger. For instance, overeating or too much caffeine are the two most common triggers. If you eat too much—especially if you eat too much animal food—or drink too much coffee, you are easily prone to angry moods. If you cut back your food consumption and eliminate meat and caffeine from your diet, you can virtually eliminate anger.

How else can you deal with anger? Any form of exercise, bodywork, or body movement technique will help, as well as visualization techniques. Solitude can help (alone, you may even yell out loud as a way to get your anger out). Or you may channel your rage through expressive arts therapy. Or try fasting—even one day can change your entire perspective.

DISTURBED SLEEP

Alcohol disrupts sleep. It blocks dreams and reduces restfulness. That's why, on the average, heavy drinkers need more sleep than nondrinkers.

Even after you quit drinking, it takes a long time before your sleep assumes a normal pattern. This will take at least a few months, or even as long as a year.

How will you be affected? You may have insomnia, or else you may have trouble getting up in the morning. Also, you will probably dream excessively.

Furthermore, many of your dreams will be extremely lucid. The most common theme for these lucid dreams? Drinking. For instance, you will dream you have lost control and taken a drink. Or you will dream you have gotten drunk and maybe landed in some kind of trouble. These dreams will bother you and you will wake with a start. The dream will seem so real, it will take you 10 or 15 minutes to realize it wasn't.

What can you do about disrupted sleep? Exercise does wonders. Daily active exercise will make you naturally tired when it's time to sleep. Doing yoga stretches at night will help you relax into a deep sleep, and doing it in the morning will cure your grogginess. These are the two favored times to do yoga. Other hints: Stop watching TV and start using relaxation techniques, such as autogenic training. Also try herbal remedies or aromatherapy.

GUILT

Most heavy drinkers experience guilt over things they've done while drunk, and usually with good reason. Very often, they have done something embarrassing, something mean, or something harmful to themselves or others.

When you stop getting drunk, you don't do all of those stupid or horrible things that made you feel guilty. So already you've made a big change.

Nevertheless, you will still feel guilty over some things. Most of this guilt will be over normal everyday affairs. Yet even this will diminish as time goes on and you start doing more and more things to feel proud about.

One thing to remember: Drop the guilt you feel for your past mistakes. Don't feel guilty for all the horrible things you did while drinking. Don't feel guilty for things you did in childhood before you started drinking. Drop it. Drop it completely. You can't change it anyway. You can only change yourself in the present, and you're doing the best you can right now.

For extra help, try "people therapies": Talk with a friend (or counselor), get into group therapy (including any recovery group), or do something for someone else. And work with your assertiveness skills, so you will not feel guilty about the way you talk to people. Or dissolve guilt with laughter. Or meditate. In meditation, you drop all thoughts of the past and of the future.

OVEREATING

When you quit any addiction, you tend to overeat. Your body replaces excesses of one thing by consuming excesses of another. When you quit drinking you will probably feel hungry all the time and you may even start overeating. This will continue for at least a few months, maybe as long as a year and a half, until your body balances itself.

One way to approach overeating: Simply allow it. Allow yourself to eat all the time, but eat only vegetables and fruit. Carry with you at all times carrot sticks, celery sticks, raisins, apples. That way, when you do overeat, you will not gain weight; in fact, you will probably lose weight.

Try fasting to adjust your internal balance. And do exercise of all kinds. Exercise burns the calories from food and helps your body digest food more efficiently.

GASTROINTESTINAL DISTRESS

When you quit drinking, it's very likely that you will experience frequent constipation or diarrhea. Or you may experience both, one alternating with the other.

Constipation is normal. It happens whenever you break an addiction to any kind of drug or food, such as alcohol, nicotine, caffeine, or sugar. It's part of your body's natural healing process. Constipation occurs as your intestinal muscles return to normal, operating on their own without the influence of whatever addictive substance you just quit.

Alcohol is one addictive substance that causes numerous health problems in the intestines. Many of these problems, such as colitis and Crohn's disease, lead to diarrhea. So after you quit drinking you will probably have diarrhea, until your body can heal itself.

How can you help the healing? Diet is one of the best ways. Eat whole grains, beans, vegetables, and fruit, all of which are high in fiber. Avoid meat, milk, and milk products, white flour products, and fruit juices. Exercise helps too. A long walk does wonders. Hatha yoga helps heal all the organs, including the intestines. You might also try a colonic to clean your intestines (no more than one or two a year), use herbal remedies, or fast to regularize your entire system.

VISIONS, HALLUCINATIONS

When you first quit drinking, you may have serious hallucinations. You know about this if you have had DTs. Hallucinations almost always accompany the convulsive shaking of DTs. People may think they see snakes or worms or insects crawling all over their bodies, for example.

These hallucinations can literally scare you to death. They can seem so real and frightening, you may do something fatal. Yet after a few days the hallucinations disappear.

Whether or not you have DTs, you may have mild hallucinations that can last for a few months after you quit drinking. What are mild hallucinations? They seem like visions. They come to you as lucid dreams, only they happen when you're awake. For instance, you may have visions of dead relatives coming back to help you. You may see religious figures reaching out to help you. Or you may envision yourself struggling to get free from some archetypal villain (such as the devil or someone from your long-ago past who was a bad influence on you).

What to do? Go with it . . . experience it. The visions and hallucinations dispel emotionally charged material stored deep within you. It's part of your long-term mental and emotional healing. So, as much as possible, take an active role in the process. You may use visualization techniques to guide your visions toward the positive. You may use affirmations to strengthen your mental imagery. You can use these to become your own guide in wonderland.

FUZZY THINKING

You may not have visions or hallucinations after you quit drinking, but you're bound to have problems with fuzzy thinking. It can last for the first two months to as long as two years after you quit. What's fuzzy thinking? It's the inability of the mind to grasp a thought or idea, resulting in confused expression and communication. It can happen with all thoughts or it can happen with specific types of thoughts.

Fuzzy thinking affects anyone who drinks alcoholically. The reason? Taken in excess, alcohol interrupts the brain's neurochemistry, interfering with thought formulation and thought transmission. When you quit drinking, it takes a long time to restore the balance of your neurochemical functioning.

But you do it. What's more, you can get your brain functioning better than it ever functioned in your entire life—even better than it functioned before you started drinking. (This applies, of course, only to the parts of your brain that still function. Any parts with physical or organic damage from alcohol abuse may remain dysfunctional.)

How can you cure fuzzy thinking? The Big Two: diet and active exercise. In diet, stay away from sugars, caffeine, nicotine, red meat, chemical additives (including artificial sugars), and any drugs, including over-the-counter drugs. Other helpful hints: Turn off the TV, try yoga, try acupuncture, massage, bodywork/body movement, fasting, intestinal cleansing, chiropractic.

THE SAME OLD FAMILY SITUATION

Quitting drinking produces another problem. When you change and your family doesn't, what happens?

Tension. Your change will be hard on family members because it means they have to change too.

By quitting drinking, you become responsible more often. You become more mature. You're less often a dependent child and less often a vicious monster. Yet people in your family have gotten used to helping the dependent child in you, or running from the vicious monster. Now what do they do?

Many marriages end when alcoholic drinkers don't change, but just as many end after drinkers quit drinking. Why? Sometimes drinkers change so much after they quit that they alienate their spouses. All of a sudden, the spouse is living with a stranger—a mature stranger, but a stranger nonetheless. And this reaction is often felt by the ex-drinker's children, parents, and extended family. The old, dependent, drunken you has died and a new you has replaced it.

What can you do to ensure your acceptance and to help those around you? Practice assertive behavior. Tell family members exactly who you are now and exactly how you feel. Give them plenty of time to accept the new you. And you need to allow them plenty of time to change their ways too. Try family counseling: it can be very effective at helping family members break out of old patterns of relating. AA can also help (AA for you, Alanon for your spouse, Alateen for your children). Other alternatives: sharing religion together, spiritual healing, "growing in love" groups, relationships training.

SEX

Excessive drinking causes sexual dysfunction in both men and women. And when you quit drinking it doesn't immediately get better. It takes time. In fact, it often gets worse before it gets better. This problem may take two months to a year to improve, depending on the seriousness of your dysfunction.

To speed healing, try yoga. It's probably the single most effective way to revitalize your sexuality. Regular physical exercise helps too. And remember to eat a good diet—one free of sugar, nicotine, and caffeine, which cause sexual problems on their own. Try also: spiritual healing, sexual relationship training, "growing in love" groups, visualization (visualize yourself a sexually healthy person).

FRIENDS

You can expect changes in your relationships with friends after you quit drinking. As with family members, anticipate that your friends will be more—or less—accepting of the new you.

When in doubt concerning your friendships, remember this important advice: Keep any friend who wishes you well after you've quit drinking and drop any friend who tries to sabotage you. The first kind of friend is a real friend. The second kind, who can't accept the nondrinking you, was never a friend in the first place.

Try to do at least as much for your friends as they do for you. That way, you will keep them. And remember to give them hugs—often.

SETBACKS

It's going to happen. Everything will be going great. You'll feel on top of the world. Then there will be some problem, an unavoidable tragedy or a serious disappointment. Your world will seem to crumble and all you'll want to do is to have a drink.

Drinking will appear as the only way you know to handle the situation. That's because it's what you've always done. Remember, you've spent a lot of time learning how to deal with problems by drinking.

Now it's time to handle these tough situations without drinking. You can learn to do it. If you do it once, you can do it again. Just practice. It gets easier over time.

Meanwhile, keep this in mind when you get hit with a setback and feel like drinking: *No matter how bad things get, you can always make them worse by drinking.*

SLIPS

Even though you know all that you know about quitting successfully, you may still slip. You may succumb to the lure of alcohol and take a drink. What happens then? What happens if you do slip and take a drink? What happens if you get drunk? What happens if you go on a binge for a week?

Catch it. Stop it. Drop the drinking and start all over again. Get right back on your own program of not drinking. Go back to Chapter 9 and pick it up from there.

Moreover, be sure to drop any guilt about making the slip. All is not lost. Look at it this way: You gained an experience. You learned something about your approach that didn't work.

It's easy enough to pick up where you left off. It's your inalienable right to continue toward your goal of becoming a nondrinker. And remember: You will be a success.

CELEBRATIONS

Many people know only one way to celebrate: have a drink. Without alcohol, how do you celebrate? How can you refuse when someone offers you champagne to celebrate a victory or raise a wedding toast? How can you refuse that beer at the end of a hard workday or turn down that martini commemorating a successful business deal?

Celebrations pose a problem because they go hand in hand with alcohol. They are also a normal part of life. You cannot escape them.

So what should you do? Find other ways to celebrate. When people raise their drinks in toast, grab your water glass instead. To celebrate a special success, have sex instead of alcohol, take a nature hike instead of drinking a beer, dance (whether there's music playing or not). Do any of your favorite alternatives to drinking (Checklist #2, Chapter 5). Do anything but drink.

Remember: You achieve more success in your life by not drinking. So don't drink to celebrate—you will only ruin your success.

If you enter into the spirit of celebration without drinking, you'll soon find that you have more fun. Allow yourself to become totally absorbed in celebrations. Instead of losing yourself in alcohol, find yourself in the celebration. And enjoy it to the fullest.

CHAPTER 12

Enjoying the Benefits of Not Drinking

Every living creature, even a puppy, is at the center of the universe.

—Anatole France

Quitting drinking is one of the best things that can happen to you. You gain many rewards: your health, your vitality, and your freedom. Now you can begin enjoying yourself.

In this chapter, you'll look on the bright side of quitting. You'll figure how much time and money you save. You'll set up a plan to give yourself rewards for not drinking. And you'll evaluate all the great benefits you gain as a result of quitting drinking.

TWO BIG BENEFITS

Most people like to hear how to save time or how to save money. How about you? When you quit drink-

276

ing, you will save both time and money. In fact, you will save a considerable amount of each.

It can be well worth it, as you'll see.

Worksheet #12

How Much Time Do You Save?

Instructions: How much time do you waste because of alcohol? Fill in the number of hours for various activities.

# of Hours   *In Average Week*

+ _____   Amount of time spent drunk.

+ _____   Time spent getting drunk. (Count only time wasted, not time when you're doing something useful; for instance, usually after the fourth or fifth drink you stop being productive.)

+ _____   Time spent making extra trips to bars to have just one drink (or two . . . or three).

+ _____   Time spent making extra trips to the liquor store or local convenience store for alcohol.

+ _____   Time spent with hangovers serious enough to keep you from doing something useful. (Include time lost from work.)

+ _____   Time spent thinking about drinking. (Time spent planning your day around alcohol, debating with yourself when to start drinking each day, planning how to pace yourself, how to hide your drinking from others, and so on.

+ _____   Time lost in nervousness as you try to postpone your first drink. Or: Time lost in physical distress as you rush to get your first drink.

# of Hours	In Average Week
+ _____	Time lost sleeping. (Alcohol causes people to need more sleep and to spend more time sleeping. After eight hours a night, count every extra hour you need as time lost due to alcohol.)
= _____	Total hours per week lost due to alcoholism (add all the above numbers).
× 52	
= _____	Numbers of hours spent in the average year on the above.
+ _____	Each year: Time spent in court hearings and in jail for alcohol-related charges, or in court-ordered driving classes.
+ _____	Each year: Time spent in hospitals due to accidents. Count accidents caused by drinking and accidents caused by hangover.
+ _____	Each year: Time spent in hospitals for medical complications of alcoholism. Count also time spent in recovery at home.
+ _____	Each year: Time spent repairing or replacing things you've damaged while drunk.
= _____ *	**Total number of hours lost each year due to alcoholism (add the five numbers above).**

* You will gain this many hours for yourself each year by quitting drinking.

Worksheet #13

How Much Money Do You Save?

Instructions: How much money do you spend on alcohol?
Fill in the dollar amount for each kind of expenditure.

Amt. Spent   *In Average Week*

+$ _____   Buying beer, wine, and liquor at liquor
               stores, supermarkets, convenience
               stores.

+$ _____   Drinking at bars (include tips).

+$ _____   Beer, wine, liquor ordered with meals at
               restaurants (include 15% for tips).

+$ _____   Amount spent on gasoline to make extra
               trips to liquor stores, bars, and so on.

+$ _____   Amount spent on taxis to take you home
               when you're drunk.

+$ _____   Amount spent buying drinks for other
               people at a bar. (Include amount to keep
               beer, wine, liquor for guests at home.)

+$ _____   Total dollars spent per week on alcohol
               habit (add all the above numbers).

× 52

=$ _____   Dollars spent in average year, on above.

+$ _____   In a year: Dollar value of items lost while
               drinking (lighters, car keys, makeup kits,
               jewelry, watches, umbrellas, hats).

+$ _____   In a year: Amount of money lost while
               drinking.

+$ _____   In a year: If you have lost your license
               due to drinking, amount spent on taxis
               and other forms of transportation to help
               you get around while you don't have
               your license.

Amt. Spent	In Average Week
+$ _____	In a year: Amount spent on fines to pay for alcohol-related legal problems. (Include amount spent for lawyers to defend you.)
+$ _____	In a year: Amount spent on alcohol-related medical problems. (Include alcohol-related injuries due to falling, getting into fights, and so on.)
+$ _____	In a year: Amount spent on things you've broken or wrecked while drunk (cars, clothing you've ruined, household items you've broken or torn up, damage due to fires you may have started while drunk).
+$ _____	In a year: Amount of income lost because you can't hold a job.
+$ _____	In a year: Amount of money lost working for a lower wage than what you're capable of earning. (Figure how much money you lose during an average year. For instance, you may be working at a job for $5 an hour, but if you stayed sober you could hold a more responsible position paying $12 an hour.)
=$ _____ *	**Total amount lost each year due to alcoholism (add the above nine numbers).**

* You will have this much extra money each year by quitting drinking.

YOU DESERVE A REWARD

You've undergone a major change: You've quit drinking. This takes a lot of strength and a lot of effort. Now, what's in it for you?

Of course you will gain some natural benefits from quitting drinking, benefits that unfold gradually, such as regaining your health, feeling better, thinking more clearly. But you deserve even more.

Studies show that rewards for success reinforce the success. That means if you reward yourself for staying off the booze, you'll want to keep up the good work. A reward gives you reason to continue.

And what could be more fun? You can choose something you really like to do . . . and do it. You can buy something special for yourself, something you always wanted. You can treat yourself to little things more often.

Don't worry about spending extra time. Don't worry about spending extra money. You have plenty of each, now that you've quit drinking. So go for it. Feel free.

Checklist #6

Claim Your Prizes

Instructions: Go through the list and choose any rewards you would like to give yourself. Write any additional ideas in the blank lines. Then plan to give yourself these rewards on a regular basis for continued success at not drinking. Give yourself at least two rewards a week—*every week*. And enjoy them.

☐ Buy yourself a book.

☐ Subscribe to a magazine you like.

☐ Buy some new running shoes, hiking shoes, work boots, or new dress shoes.

☐ Buy yourself some new clothing (a dress, a pair of slacks, a new hat).

☐ Buy some new fishing equipment.

- [ ] Buy a new record, tape, or compact disc.
- [ ] Buy yourself a new set of work tools, a special power tool you've always wanted, or a new work bench.
- [ ] Buy some new camera equipment.
- [ ] Buy yourself a special piece of equipment to help with any hobby. Ideas:
  - [ ] An easel for art.
  - [ ] A pottery wheel.
  - [ ] A typewriter or word processor.

_____

_____

_____

- [ ] Write a poem.
- [ ] Get together with a friend.
- [ ] Go to a movie.
- [ ] Go out dancing.
- [ ] Go to a comedy club for an evening of laughter.
- [ ] Go out to dinner.
- [ ] Get a massage.
- [ ] Take a long walk.
- [ ] Take a special class.
- [ ] Get your hair styled.
- [ ] Listen to a piece of music.
- [ ] Read a book or magazine.
- [ ] Make a special meal.
- [ ] Call a friend for a long chat.
- [ ] Take a long bath with herbal bath oils.
- [ ] Take some time all to yourself to work on a craft or hobby you like.
- [ ] Take time to work on your favorite creative project (painting, sculpting, writing, music, photography).
- [ ] Work with any of the healing techniques you liked in Worksheet #7 (Chapter 8). You can go to a specialist, take classes, or study on your own. Write what you will do (for instance: "go for acupuncture treatments once a week").

☐   Other rewards you would like (for ideas, see Chapter
     5, Checklist #2, Alternatives to Drinking):

Treat yourself. You deserve it.

HAVING FUN

Have you noticed? Now that you've quit drinking,
things are changing. You're beginning to grow. You're
beginning to feel better. Life suddenly seems worth-
while.

Have you seen the changes?

Generally, you become more responsible. You feel
happier, healthier, more optimistic. You begin to
think more clearly, show and receive more love,
know more, become wiser and more mature. In short,
your life is more successful.

How have you changed? Take a good look. Use the
following worksheet as a guide.

Worksheet #14

The Benefits of Not Drinking

Instructions: Put a check next to the changes you've made and benefits you've been enjoying by not drinking. Consider how important these changes and these benefits are to you. Remember them. Write them on a separate piece of paper and review them from time to time. Remind yourself over and over that the only way to get these benefits is to stay off the alcohol.

- ☐ I'm getting healthy again.
- ☐ I have my health for the first time in my life.
- ☐ I don't have as many headaches.
- ☐ I don't have as many physical pains.
- ☐ My liver is healing (no pains in my right side anymore).
- ☐ My pancreas is healing (no pains in my left side anymore).
- ☐ My stomach isn't always hurting.
- ☐ My stomach isn't upset as often.
- ☐ My ulcer is going away.
- ☐ My intestines are getting stronger.
- ☐ My bowel movements are becoming regular again.
- ☐ My blood pressure is becoming normal.
- ☐ My heart feels stronger (my chest pains are going away).
- ☐ My eyes are healing. I can see more clearly.
- ☐ I feel more limber.
- ☐ My muscles don't ache as much.
- ☐ I'm beginning to eat normally again.
- ☐ I'm beginning to lose weight and look more trim.
- ☐ My nerves are settling down. I'm not as nervous or tense anymore.
- ☐ I don't get angry as often.

- [ ] I don't get as angry as I used to.
- [ ] I don't feel violent anymore.
- [ ] I feel stronger inside.
- [ ] Sex is better.
- [ ] I can now have healthier babies.
- [ ] My concentration is better.
- [ ] My creativity is returning.
- [ ] I can think more clearly.
- [ ] My memory has returned.
- [ ] I feel good about myself.
- [ ] I'm getting more compliments from others.
- [ ] I look better physically.
- [ ] I'm getting to work on time.
- [ ] I feel confident I can hold a job now.
- [ ] I feel comfortable driving. I don't have to worry about tickets, lawyers, fines, losing my license.
- [ ] I can go out and have a good time without making a fool of myself.
- [ ] It feels good not having to sneak drinks anymore.
- [ ] I feel more open than I used to.
- [ ] I feel like I can be more honest with people, including myself.
- [ ] I don't complain as much as I used to.
- [ ] I feel like I'm beginning to grow . . . like maybe my life can go somewhere now.
- [ ] I no longer feel like a loser.
- [ ] I have more money to spend on the things I want.
- [ ] I have a stronger sense of pride and accomplishment.
- [ ] I feel like I can make something out of myself and I'm beginning to do so.
- [ ] I feel more organized now.
- [ ] I trust myself and my own judgment more.
- [ ] I don't feel as guilty about my behavior anymore.
- [ ] I'm more assertive now.

☐ I can communicate better.

☐ More and more, I can be around other people and feel comfortable with them.

☐ I'm less anxious.

☐ I feel more loving.

☐ I'm much better with my family.

☐ I'm resolving issues with my family.

☐ Now I go out more often with my family.

☐ I now have a more positive view about relationships with the opposite sex.

☐ My relationship with a sexual partner is getting better.

☐ My loving relationships are getting better.

☐ Relationships with my friends are getting better.

☐ More people seem to like me now.

☐ I feel I can help others in certain ways, and I'm beginning to do so.

☐ In general, my life gets better and better.

☐ Lately, I'm enjoying myself more and more.

CHAPTER 13

Inspirations to Help Make Quitting Easy

The great art of life is how to turn the surplus life of the soul into life for the body.
—*Henry David Thoreau*

Here, you'll find music for the soul, harmonies of thoughts and feelings to help awaken your deep inner self. These are personal meditations—ideas that you can act on—to make your life go easier.

What's an inspiration?

Inspiration literally means to breathe in. Each new breath bursts with oxygen, energy, vitality. Breath continues life itself. Breath is soul-life, the life of the spirit.

Here are ten inspirations. Each can be extremely helpful for anyone quitting drinking.

DO ONE THING AT A TIME

People who have quit drinking often feel overwhelmed with too much to do. Their minds constantly juggle thoughts of five, ten, fifteen things they have to do. They can't even do one thing well because, while trying to do one thing, their minds remain preoccupied with something else.

What can you do about this? Change your approach. Drop everything from your mind but the thing at hand. Concentrate on the immediate task. Center every ounce of your attention on it.

If your mind begins to wander, stop. Stop everything. For example, let's say you're trying to read something and your mind is thinking a hundred different things. Stop. Stop your reading immediately. Tell your mind, "Okay, you want to think about these hundred different things . . . I'll give you five minutes . . . then I want your entire attention focused on this article I'm reading." Give the mind five minutes. Listen to all the thoughts. Take each thought one at a time, thoughts about dishes not getting done, about why you're not working at a higher-paying job, about guilt over some inadvertent statement you made to a friend last week, about getting the lawn mowed, about some sexual need you have. Give each thought its due, until you've reviewed your entire mental list of distractions. Then get back to your reading.

Practice paying attention. Focus your mind. One way: Practice batting away all thoughts that interfere. Visualize yourself using a baseball bat to knock each intruding thought out of your mind.

Do one thing at a time. If you're going to eat, eat. If you're going to talk, talk. If you're going to hammer a nail, hammer a nail. Do nothing else but the thing at hand. You'll get much more done that way and have far better results.

ALL THINGS COME TO THOSE WHO WAIT

This saying comes from the East; in the West, we say, "Patience is a virtue." Both mean the same—except the Eastern saying more aptly describes what you need to do.

You need to wait. It's something you must learn.

You may want a lot of things in your life. And you may want many things right now. Indeed, you may get impatient waiting for things to happen. But if you try to force things to happen, you will not succeed. You cannot get what you want by forcing.

Deep inside, you must be ready for changes. It takes time. You must be mature enough in your life to handle certain kinds of benefits, including financial success.

If you learn to wait for what you want, you will work toward it gradually and change accordingly. Then one day it will happen. It will come to you. The thing you have wanted, and waited for, will be yours.

So relax. Be patient. And wait.

OLD ENDINGS ARE NEW BEGINNINGS

As one thing ends, something new begins. This is true of everything in the universe, including everything inside of you.

So as you change, drop the old, make way for the new. Remember to leave the past in the past. Open yourself to the new. Don't linger over losses; consider what you're gaining.

As one thing ends, get ready for your adventure. Something new will soon begin. The moment of discovery awaits.

EVERYTHING CHANGES

Everything changes all the time. Nothing remains the same—even for a moment. Realize this and you can go with it, instead of fighting it.

Whenever we resist change, whenever we refuse to change, we stagnate. Inside we become stuck, brittle, unhealthy. But the more we go with changes, the more we allow ourselves to change, the more we grow. Experiencing changes, we renew ourselves, we refresh ourselves, we become wise.

So be flexible in your life. Allow yourself to change. Go with the flow. Meditate on change itself until, through meditation, you become one with the ever-changing world around you.

DON'T TAKE ANYTHING
TOO SERIOUSLY

This so-called universe appears as a juggling, a picture show. To be happy, look upon it so.
—*Tantric saying*

Nothing in this universe has much meaning beyond what the mind sees in it. Actually, the mind attaches too much meaning to things. Relax the mind and the world changes.

At best, we get only glimpses of reality in our lives, fleeting moments of meaning. When allowed, the mind can just as easily find no meaning. At any given moment, one thing may seem true, yet the opposite may also seem true.

When you look at the world on one level, you might see meaning. When you look at the world on another level, you might see no meaning at all. But when you view the world on both levels at the same time, you may well burst out in laughter.

LIVE THIS VERY MOMENT

How do you know what's happening now? Think about it and you lose it. Why? Too many thoughts clutter your vision.

Try this: Drop all thoughts of the future. Drop all thoughts of the past. Say nothing to yourself. Form no sentences, no words. What's left? Receptivity to all that's around you. Oneness . . . you become one with the world each and every moment.

Here's a simple practice: Choose anything (the grass, the sky, a tree, anything you like). Meditate on it; become one with it. Allow yourself to merge with it and it to merge with you. Feel it fully. Now notice that your mind is still. If your mind so much as says a word, you lose the moment. If your mind says "green," you lose the grass.

This is what meditation is all about—quieting the mind. The mind chatters on and on, endlessly. If you can drop your mind, you can gain the moment. By opening yourself in this way, each moment feels infinite.

Now consider this (from William Blake):

To see a World in a Grain of Sand
And a Heaven in a Wild Flower,
Hold Infinity in the palm of your hand
And Eternity in an hour.

YOU CAN'T HAVE EVERYTHING
ALL AT ONCE

People want things, many things. We all desire something more than what we have. Yet desire causes pain. Why? Because you desire only things you don't have. That means you feel a lack, something missing. And that causes pain.

Desire means you feel incomplete. You need something more. Ideally, you would like to have everything all at once. It would make you feel complete. Yet you can't have everything all at once. It's impossible. It can never happen. You will always want something more.

The root of the problem is desire itself. So here's what to do: Drop desire. Stop wanting more and more. Drop it. It is desire that hurts. It is that need for something more that makes you feel incomplete.

You don't need the new sports car, the new love, the hundred thousand dollars, the new pair of shoes, to make you feel complete. Drop your desires and you will feel whole the way you are. One person . . . one integrity.

HEAR THE TRUTH WITHIN

Open yourself to the inner sanctum. Open yourself to your body. Go inside and listen to what your body tells you and be sensitive to every detail. Don't get stuck in your mind. Remember, the brain is one of many organs in your body. When you need to think, use this organ. Otherwise, don't think. Just feel.

Inside, your body holds incredible wisdom and it's up to you to discover it. How can you do that? Become quiet with yourself. Become your body. Hear your body from deep within and let it tell you what you need.

YOUR LIFE IS AS LONG AS YOU WANT IT TO BE

When you quit drinking, your life opens up to you. Totally. No longer does your life seem to be a whirlwind affair, passing you by.

When you quit, it seems like time slows down. You begin living more in every moment. Consequently, your whole life seems to transcend time. You begin to feel as if you're living in eternity.

Life has no boundaries now. You will live longer in actual number of years . . . and be in better health. In fact, the more attention you pay to your health, the more years you will add to your life.

But now each moment of your life feels limitless. Each moment feels vast, greater than the moments you've known before. Now, as the moments grow long, your life is as long as you want it to be.

YOU CAN HAVE THIS DAY FOR FREE

Let's face it. On certain days, things go wrong. On some days everything seems to go wrong.

What can you do? Simply write it off. Things will be better tomorrow, or the next day. But today, don't worry. You can have this day for free.

Already you've gained a hundred days a hundred ways. Simply by quitting drinking you've added years to your life. Plus, by taking good care of yourself and improving your health, you'll add extra days to your life on a regular basis.

Yes, you will live longer.

So now—whenever you need to—take a free day. Just give yourself the day. Allow the day to go any way it will. Don't even worry if nothing gets done. If you're having a bad day, write it off. If you simply need a break, take it. Either way, just let the day go in utter happiness. You'll have another day to make up for it.

CHAPTER 14

Making Your Life a Success

> *"Would you tell me, please, which way I ought to go from here?"*
>
> *"That depends a good deal on where you want to get to," said the Cat.*
>
> *"I don't much care where—" said Alice.*
>
> *"Then it doesn't matter which way you go," said the Cat.*
>
> *"—so long as I get somewhere," Alice added as an explanation.*
>
> *"Oh, you're sure to do that," said the Cat, "if only you walk long enough."*
>
> —*Lewis Carroll*, Alice's Adventures in Wonderland

Here's your big payoff. You have made major changes. You have fought a long, hard battle. You may even have gone through great difficulties to get here. But you have won.

Now you're starting to control your own life. Indeed, your life has become more manageable than ever. And because of this, you can raise your sights. Now you can pick your own goals and achieve them.

If you apply the right amount of effort, you can achieve almost any goal you choose.

WHAT ARE YOUR IMPORTANT GOALS?

The more you reclaim your life from alcohol (and other addictions), the more you can achieve. By dropping your addictions, you become stronger and more in control of your life. Success is then more likely.

It doesn't happen all at once. It happens in steps. By quitting alcohol, you take a giant step toward personal growth and improvement. By quitting other addictions (drugs, nicotine, caffeine, sugar, overeating), you gain even more power. As you clear away these obstacles, your life transforms miraculously and success becomes inevitable.

What do you choose to do? Think about it. It's good to know what you want, what you're aiming for. How can you hit a target if you can't see it? In Worksheet #15, you'll list some goals that are important to you. Then, at the end of this chapter, you'll learn specific ways to achieve these goals.

Worksheet #15

Personal Life Goals

Instructions: Write your personal goals. Be realistic. For each type of goal, write what you'd like to accomplish in one year, in five years, in your lifetime. Take your time. If you're not sure of your goals in a specific area, come back to it later. Describe your goals as you see them today. But remember, your goals will probably change over time, so review this chart regularly and revise as necessary.

Types of goals	One-year goal	Five-year goal	Lifetime goal
Physical			
• physical appearance	_____	_____	_____
• health	_____	_____	_____
Mental			
• clarity	_____	_____	_____
• creativity	_____	_____	_____
• attitude	_____	_____	_____
Emotional			
• calmness	_____	_____	_____
• happiness	_____	_____	_____
• self-confidence	_____	_____	_____
Spiritual			
• renewed faith	_____	_____	_____
• inner peace	_____	_____	_____
Social			
• strangers	_____	_____	_____
• acquaintances	_____	_____	_____
• friends	_____	_____	_____
Family			
• spouse	_____	_____	_____
• children	_____	_____	_____
• mother	_____	_____	_____
• brother(s)	_____	_____	_____
• sister(s)	_____	_____	_____

Types of goals	One-year goal	Five-year goal	Lifetime goal
Career			
• job	_____	_____	_____
• business venture	_____	_____	_____
Financial	_____	_____	_____
Education	_____	_____	_____
Sports/fitness	_____	_____	_____
Diet	_____	_____	_____
Hobbies	_____	_____	_____
Community service	_____	_____	_____
Other: _____	_____	_____	_____

GETTING WHAT YOU WANT AND GETTING GOOD RESULTS WITHOUT ALCOHOL

At this moment you are in a very good position. By quitting drinking, you have proven yourself capable of achieving a goal. That means you have dealt with, and overcome, obstacles along the way. But that's not all. Now that you've quit drinking, you have gotten rid of a major obstacle that has prevented you from achieving important life goals.

In Worksheet #15, you listed personal life goals that are important to you. That's the beginning, because once you know your goals, you can begin doing what's necessary to achieve them. So what's necessary?

Zig Ziglar, renowned teacher of goal achievement, travels the country giving dynamic talks on goal achievement and how to be a winner. (Some of Zig's talks have been videotaped and are available from Nightingale-Conant Corporation at 800–525–9000. I recommend you order the one titled *Goals*.) Zig presents seven steps to achieving goals. They are:

1. Identify your goal.
2. Set a deadline.
3. List obstacles you must overcome.
4. Identify people who can help and get them to help you.
5. List the skills you need to accomplish your goal. Obtain these skills.
6. Develop a plan and write it down.
7. List the benefits of achieving your goal.

Now write your seven steps for each goal you listed in Worksheet #15. Then follow the steps. Start following your plan for each of your goals. By working toward your goals in this manner, you will be successful.

CHAPTER 15

Freedom

I only ask to be free. The butterflies are free.
—*Charles Dickens*

A h, freedom . . . what we won't do to get it . . . but
how easy it is to lose.

Alcohol takes your freedom away. Chained to the
bottle, you can hardly go anywhere without being
concerned about your alcohol supply. Some alcoholic
drinkers can't even go to the movies without carrying
along a half-pint.

Deep in the addiction, your whole life becomes
tied to alcohol. You can't even get up in the morning
or wake up in the middle of the night without needing
a drink. In the first case you need alcohol to wake you
up; in the second case you need alcohol to put you
back to sleep.

At this stage of addiction, alcohol controls you.
You're stuck. It's like half your life is gone; whole
parts of you are no longer available to you. It's like
half of you is already dead and buried.

That's why everybody addicted to alcohol, deep
down inside, wants to quit. The reasons are clear.
Quitting drinking sets you free. Quitting drinking
makes you whole again. Quitting drinking gives you

new breath, new life, new hope for happiness. What more could you ask for?

FEELING FREE

Life changes when you quit drinking. Have you noticed? You've become free, perhaps freer than you've ever known. But along with freedom comes responsibility.

With alcohol, you were often irresponsible. Many basic responsibilities—keeping a job, meeting the needs of your family, meeting your own needs, treating other people with respect, and so on—were just too much for you. What's worse, you even used alcohol as an excuse: "I couldn't help it; I just drank too much."

Now you have no excuses. Now you're out in the open, on your own. How do you handle the responsibility?

Easy. Simply get right into it.

You have just reclaimed a big part of your life. Now it's time to live and watch how things change. When you become so completely involved in every aspect of your life, you begin enjoying it fully. Life's responsibilities soon become life's pleasures.

You begin to like your work—even if it takes changing your job—and you begin to succeed at it. You feel good about meeting the needs of your family, especially their emotional needs. You begin to feel good about yourself as you regain your health. And you begin to enjoy other people. You start showing respect for other people and, the big reward, they start respecting you.

So how do you deal with open spaces? Step right in. Do what's needed. Once in a while, do something silly just for fun. Stay with your program but, above all, enjoy yourself.

STEERING CLEAR OF TROUBLE

> *To free oneself is nothing; it is being free that is hard.*
>
> —*André Gide*

If you stay goal-directed and keep working toward your goals, you'll maintain your freedom. Sure, you can take a day off once in a while, but nearly every day you need to work toward your goals.

Does this sound like a grind? Like there's no fun involved? Maybe it sounds hard, but remember, when you achieve your goals you gain many benefits and rewards. For instance, if one of your goals is to lose weight, you'll begin hearing compliments from other people, you'll begin feeling better inside, you'll enjoy greater health, you'll live longer. Losing weight may be work, it may even be hard work, but the benefits are worth it.

So keep your perspective on things. And keep your course.

Practice #9

Three Ways to Keep Your Freedom

Do these three things to help maintain your freedom:

- **Keep rewarding yourself.** Give yourself gifts, rewards and prizes on a regular basis (at least one every two weeks). To find something new or to recall your favorite rewards, go over Checklist #6 in Chapter 12.
- **Review your benefits again and again.** Over the course of your life, you continually gain new and different benefits by not drinking. Knowing these benefits helps you stay off the booze. So review your list (Worksheet #14, Chapter 12) often, maybe every two months, and add to it, as necessary.
- **Check your life goals regularly.** Review your progress toward these goals. As you achieve them, write down the benefits you experience. Have your goals changed? If so, revise Worksheet #15, Chapter 14. Review your goals and your progress toward your goals on a regular basis, maybe twice a month.

A NEW YOU

Who are you now? Without alcohol changing your body chemistry, don't you feel like a different person? Aren't you more mature . . . more capable . . . more kind . . . more loving?

Yes. You are.

Of course you will have some days when you feel bad. But keep in mind the fact that they will pass. Overall you keep gaining ground, changing inside, discovering something new about yourself.

In fact, when you quit drinking you assume a new identity. You start becoming someone new. Indeed, the transformation is so complete, you actually become a different person.

So go with it. Get yourself up to it. Enjoy the changes and enjoy the new you.

For fun you may even want to change your name. It may be something as simple as asking to be called Michael instead of Mike or Susan instead of Susie. Tell your family and friends. You will probably want to get rid of any drinking nicknames. For example, you may prefer Bill to Kid Chaleen, Don over Wild Man, Jack instead of Moon. Or you may want to choose a brand-new name—maybe even something personally important or symbolic to you.

Meanwhile, you may or may not want to call yourself an "alcoholic." If you decide not to refer to yourself as an alcoholic, that's fine. For practical purposes, you're not an alcoholic when you're not drinking. On the other hand, you may prefer to call yourself an alcoholic or a "recovering alcoholic" because it gives you a constant reminder that you cannot drink. That's fine too, as it serves a useful purpose.

Whatever your choice, be sure to acknowledge the new you. Open yourself to a changing pattern. Drop the old alcoholic part of you. Let the new you shine through.

In the old self, you were constrained. In the new self, you are open to all the world. In the old self, alcohol kept you locked in a box. In the new self, someone has opened the box. And now . . . you're free.

Indeed, you have opened the box yourself. You have quit drinking on your own and you deserve a great deal of praise. You have become a success to yourself and to many other people around you.

Good work.

Keep it up.

Afterword

Congratulations.

You have shown the courage to change. At times it wasn't easy. But you have worked hard and you have become a success. You deserve a great amount of credit.

Now you can begin enjoying your life more fully. You've grown. You've opened the door to many additional opportunities, and you feel you have more choices in your life than ever. You've gained your freedom.

I encourage you to continue your success. I feel certain you can—and I feel confident you will.

Now, if you have a moment, I'd like to hear from you. Over the years, I've conducted hundreds of interviews with folks who had problems with drinking. I've developed what I think is the best program to meet everybody's needs. But tell me, how well did the program work for you? What methods worked best? What ideas do you have to help me improve this book?

On the other hand, if you want help with a specific problem, or if you want me to answer any questions you may have, I'm available. I'll send a response as soon as possible.

Please write to me:

Jerry Dorsman
c/o New Dawn
551 Elk Mills Road, Box 71
Elk Mills, MD 21920

Bibliography and Recommended Reading

AA World Services. *Alcoholics Anonymous.* New York: Alcoholics Anonymous Publishing, 1955.

———. *Alcoholics Anonymous Comes of Age.* New York: Harper, 1957.

———. *Comments on AA's Triennial Surveys.* New York: AA World Services, 1990.

Addiction & Recovery Magazine. Cleveland, OH: International Publishing Group (1990–1993: many issues, many articles). Formerly *Alcoholism and Addiction Magazine.*

Airola, Paavo, ND, Ph.D. *Hypoglycemia: A Better Approach.* Phoenix, AZ: Health Plus Publishers, 1977.

Alberti, Robert, Ph.D., and Emmons, Michael, Ph.D. *Your Perfect Right: A Guide to Assertive Living* (6th ed.). San Luis Obispo, CA: Impact Publishers, 1990.

Alcoholism and Addiction Magazine. Cleveland, OH: Quantum Publishing Co. (many issues, many articles). Also: *Recovery Magazine* (published as insert to *Alcoholism and Addiction Magazine*).

American Lung Association. *Freedom from Smoking in 20 Days.* American Lung Association, 1980.

Anderson, Bob. *Stretching.* Bolinas, CA: Shelter Publications, 1980.

Annand, Margo. *The Art of Sexual Ecstasy.* Los Angeles: Jeremy P. Tarcher, 1989.

Barrett, Clarence, JD. *Beyond AA: Dealing Responsibly with Alcohol.* Greenleaf, OR: Positive Attitudes, 1991.

Beasley, Joseph D., MD. *How to Defeat Alcoholism: Nutritional Guidelines for Getting Sober.* New York: Times Books, 1989.

———. *Wrong Diagnosis, Wrong Treatment.* New York: Essential Medical Information, 1987.

Bufe, Charles. *Alcoholics Anonymous: Cult or Cure?* San Francisco: See Sharp Press, 1991.

Burgess, Louise Bailey. *Alcohol and Your Health.* Los Angeles: Charles Publishing, 1973.

Burns, John (and three other recovered alcoholics). *The Answer to Addiction.* New York: Harper & Row, 1975.

Buscaglia, Leo F. *Love.* New York: Ballantine Books, 1982.

Chafetz, Morris, MD. *Why Drinking Can Be Good for You.* New York: Stein and Day, 1976.

Chang, Jolan. *The Tao of Love and Sex.* London: Wildwood House, 1977.

Christopher, James. *Unhooked: Staying Sober and Drug-free.* Buffalo: Prometheus Books, 1989.

———. *SOS Sobriety: The Proven Alternative to 12-Step Programs.* Buffalo: Prometheus Books, 1992.

Colbin, Annemarie. *Food and Healing.* New York: Ballantine Books, 1986.

The Counselor Magazine. Arlington, VA: National

Association of Alcoholism & Drug Abuse Counselors (NAADAC) (many issues, many articles).

Cousens, Gabriel, MD. "Living Food." *New Frontier Magazine*, September 1989.

Dennison, Darwin; Prevet, Thomas, and Affleck, Michael. *Alcohol and Behavior*. St. Louis: Mosby, 1980.

Denzin, Norman K. *The Alcoholic Self*. Newbury Park, CA: Sage Publications, 1987.

———. *The Recovering Alcoholic*. Newbury Park, CA: Sage, 1987.

Desmond, Edward. "Out in the Open." *Time Magazine*, Nov. 30, 1987.

Douglas, Nik, and Slinger, Penny. *Sexual Secrets*. New York: Destiny Books, 1979.

Dufty, William. *Sugar Blues*. New York: Warner Books, 1976.

Edwards, Griffith, and Grant, Marcus (editors). *Alcoholism Treatment in Transition*. Baltimore: University Park Press, 1980.

Employee Assistance Magazine. Waco, TX: Stevens Publishing Corp. (many issues: many articles).

Esko, Edward and Esko, Wendy. *Macrobiotic Cooking for Everyone*. Tokyo: Japan Publications, 1980.

Fields, Rick with Taylor, Peggy; Weyler, Rex, and Ingrasci, Rick. *Chop Wood, Carry Water: A Guide to Finding Spiritual Fulfillment in Everyday Life*. Los Angeles: Tarcher, 1984.

Finnegan, John, and Gray, Daphne. *Recovery from Addiction*. Berkeley, CA: Celestial Arts, 1990.

Folan, Lilias M. *Lilias, Yoga and You*. New York: Bantam Books, 1972.

Foster, Fred. *The Alcohol Trap*. Wheaton, IL: Tyndale House Publishers, 1982.

Foundation for Inner Peace. *A Course in Miracles*. Tiburon, CA: Foundation for Inner Peace, 1975.

Galanter, Marc, MD; Egelko, Susan, Ph.D., and Edwards, Helen, MPH. "Rational Recovery: Alternative to AA for Addiction," *American Journal of Drug & Alcohol Abuse*: 19 (4), pp. 499–510 (1993).

Hackl, John R., and Hackl, Alphons J. *The Way Out of Alcoholism*. Washington, DC: Acropolis Books, 1984.

Health Education Center of Maryland Department of Health and Mental Hygiene. *Getting Fit Your Way: A Self-Paced Fitness Guide*. Washington, DC: U.S. Government Printing Office, 1983.

Hoskins, Ray. *Rational Madness: The Paradox of Addiction*. Blue Ridge Summit, PA: Tab Books, 1989.

Israel, Yedy, and Mardones, Jorge (editors). *The Biological Basis of Alcoholism*. New York: Wiley-Interscience, 1971.

Jampolsky, Gerald. *Love Is Letting Go of Fear*. New York: Bantam, 1981.

Johnson, Vernon E. *I'll Quit Tomorrow*. New York: Harper & Row, 1973.

Kaminer, Wendy. *I'm Dysfunctional, You're Dysfunctional: The Recovery Movement and Other Self-Help Fashions*. Reading, MA: Addison-Wesley, 1992.

Ketcham, Katherine, and Mueller, L. Ann, MD. *Eating Right to Live Sober*. New York: New American Library, 1983.

Kirkpatrick, Jean, Ph.D. *Goodbye Hangovers, Hello Life*. New York: Atheneum, 1986.

———. *Turnabout: New Help for the Woman Alcoholic*. New York: Bantam, 1977.

Kotzsch, Ron. "Are Your Compulsions Out of Control?" *EastWest Journal*, June 1983.

Kurtz, Ernest. *Not-God: A History of Alcoholics Anonymous*. Center City, MN: Hazelden Educational Services, 1979. (Reprinted as *AA: The Story*, San Francisco: Harper, 1988.)

Leviton, Richard. "Staying Drugfree Naturally." *East-West Journal*, March 1988.

Mathews-Larsen, Joan, Ph.D. *Alcoholism, The Biochemical Connection: A Breakthrough Seven-Week Self-Treatment Program*. New York: Villard Books, 1992.

Maultsby, Maxie C., MD. *A Million Dollars for Your Hangover: The Illustrated Guide for the New Self-Help Treatment Method*. Lexington, KY: Rational Self-Help Books, 1978.

Maxwell, Ruth. *The Booze Battle*. New York: Ballantine Books, 1977.

McLanahan, Amrita Sandra, MD. *Health, Yoga and Anatomy* (videotape). Buckingham, VA: Integral Yoga Distribution, Satchidananda Ashram.

Milam, Dr. James R., and Ketcham, Katherine. *Under the Influence: A Guide to the Myths and Realities of Alcoholism*. Seattle: Madrona Publishers, 1981.

Miller, Dr. William R. (editor). *The Addictive Behaviors: Treatment of Alcoholism, Drug Abuse, Smoking, and Obesity*. New York: Pergamon Press, 1980.

———. "The Effectiveness of Alcoholism Treatment Modalities." *Testimony to the U.S. Senate Committee on Governmental Affairs*, June 16, 1988.

Miller, Dr. William R., and Muñoz, Ricardo F. *How to Control Your Drinking*. Albuquerque: University of New Mexico Press, 1982.

Mindell, Earl. *Earl Mindell's Vitamin Bible*. New York: Rawson, Wade, 1979.

Mooney, Al J., MD; Eisenberg, Arlene, and Eisneberg, Howard. *The Recovery Book*. New York: Workman, 1992.

Mueller, L. Ann, MD, and Ketcham, Katherine. *Re-*

covering: *How to Get and Stay Sober*. New York: Bantam, 1987.

Mumey, Jack, and Hatcher, Anne S., Ed.D., RD. *Good Food for a Sober Life: A Diet and Nutrition Book for Recovering Alcoholics and Those Who Love Them*. Chicago: Contemporary Books, 1987.

Muramoto, Naboru, with Abehsera, Michel. *Healing Ourselves*. New York: Avon, 1973.

Myers, Judy, with Mellin, Maribeth. *Staying Sober*. New York: Congdon & Weed, 1987.

Null, Gary, and Null, Steven. *How to Get Rid of the Poisons in Your Body*. New York: Arco, 1977.

O'Keefe, Rip, Ph.D. *Sober Living Workbook*. Center City, MN: Hazelden, 1980.

Orford, Jim. *Excessive Appetites: A Psychological View of Addiction*. New York: Wiley, 1985.

Ott, John. *Health and Light*. New York: Pocket Books, 1976.

Patterson, James, and Kim, Peter. *The Day America Told the Truth*. New York: Prentice Hall, 1991.

Patterson, Meg, MBE, MBChB, FRCSE. *Hooked? NET: The New Approach to Drug Cure*. London: Faber and Faber, 1986.

Peele, Stanton (editor). *Visions of Addiction*. Lexington, MA: D.C. Heath, 1988.

Peele, Stanton, Ph.D., and Brodsky, Archie, with Arnold, Mary. *The Truth About Addiction and Recovery: The Life Process Program for Outgrowing Destructive Habits*. New York: Simon & Schuster, 1991.

Perez, Joseph F., Ph.D. *Alcoholism: Causes, Effects, and Treatment*. Muncie, IN: Accelerated Development, 1992.

Phelps, Janice K., MD, and Nourse, Alan E., MD. *The Hidden Addiction and How to Get Free*. Boston: Little, Brown, 1986.

Plagenhoef, Richard L., MD, and Adler, Carol. *Why Am I Still Addicted?: A Holistic Approach to Recovery*. Blue Ridge Summit, PA: Tab Books, 1992.

Porth, Carol. *Pathophysiology: Concepts of Altered Health States*. Philadelphia: J.B. Lippincott, 1982.

Pritikin, Nathan, with McGrady, Patrick Jr. *The Pritikin Program for Diet and Exercise*. New York: Grosset & Dunlap, 1979.

Professional Counselor Magazine. Redmond, WA: A&D Publications Corp. (many issues, many articles).

Rajneesh, Bhagwan Shree. *The Book of Secrets* (5 volumes). New York: Harper & Row, 1974.

Ray, Sondra. *Loving Relationships*. Berkeley, CA: Celestial Arts, 1980.

Robertson, Dr. Joel. *Help Yourself: A Revolutionary Alternative Recovery Program*. Nashville: Thomas Nelson Publishers, 1992.

Robinson, Corrine, and Lawler, Marilyn. *Normal and Theraputic Nutrition* (16th ed.). New York: Macmillan, 1982.

Rogers, Jacquelyn. *You Can Stop: A SmokEnder Approach to Quitting Smoking and Sticking to It*. New York: Simon & Schuster, 1977.

Royce, James E. *Alcohol Problems and Alcoholism: A Comprehensive Survey*. New York: Free Press, 1981.

Saifer, Phyllis, MD, MPH, and Zellerbach, Merla. *Detox*. New York: Ballantine Books, 1984.

Selvig, Dick, and Riley, Don. *High & Dry*. Blue Earth, MN: Piper Press, 1980.

Seymour, Richard, and Smith, David, MD. *Drugfree: A Unique, Positive Approach to Staying Off Alcohol and Other Drugs*. Facts on File, 1987.

Siegel, Bernie. *Love, Medicine & Miracles*. New York: Harper & Row, 1986.

Smith, Manuel J. *When I Say No, I Feel Guilty*. New York: Bantam, 1975.

Steiner, Claude. *Healing Alcoholism*. New York: Grove Press, 1979.

Tierra, Michael, GA, ND. *The Way of Herbs*. New York: Washington Square Press, 1980.

Tracy, Lisa. *The Gradual Vegetarian*. New York: Dell, 1985.

Trimpey, Jack. *The Small Book: A Revolutionary Alternative for Overcoming Alcohol and Drug Dependence*. New York: Delacorte, 1992.

Tortera, Gerald; Funke, Berdell, and Case, Christine. *Microbiology: An Introduction*. Menlo Park, CA: Benjamin/Cummings, 1982.

Vaughan, Clark. *Addictive Drinking: The Road to Recovery for Problem Drinkers and Those Who Love Them*. New York: Viking Press, 1982.

Williams, Dr. Roger J. *The Prevention of Alcoholism Through Nutrition*. New York: Bantam, 1981.

Winters, Ariel. *Alternatives for the Problem Drinker: AA Is Not the Only Way*. New York: Drake Publishers, 1978.

Ziglar, Zig. *Goals* (videotape). Chicago: Nightingale Conant Corporation, 1986.

Index

Acetaldehyde, 22, 24, 31
Acupuncture, 193–195
Affirmations, 201–202, 203
Afterword, 305–306
Alcohol
  addiction, 18–30, 34–35, 95
  and brain neurochemistry,
      20–22, 31, 271
  as food, 21, 35
  as friend, 105
  as medicine, 19, 30
  as sedative, 21, 26, 29, 31
  as toxin, 20, 24, 26, 27, 30
  calories of, 21, 35
  conversion to sugar, 21
  damage caused by, 20–21, 30,
      51–52, 61–69
  detox, 69–70
  freedom from, 300–304
  your relationship to, 50, 51,
      256–258
Alcoholics Anonymous
  how AA can help, 81–84, 230,
      236
  membership, 81, 83
  problems with AA, 1, 3, 82,
      84–89
  religious methodology of, 81,
      85–86
  success rate, 1, 82, 222
  trying a few meetings, 84
  your choice about, 89–90
Alcoholism
  a dietary disease, 30–35
  a learned behavior, 12–14
  a non-alcoholic part of you,
      14–16

a personal struggle, 16–18
a physical addiction, 18–30
a way of coping, 10–12, 52
as block to spiritual growth, 236
as habit, 93
as need for physical affection,
    233
costs, 2
in teenagers, 2, 26
medical problems caused by,
    61–69
statistics, 2–3
violence and death rates, 2–3, 20
Alcoholic drinking
  alternatives to, 106–112
  causing death, 57–58
  definition, 30, 38
Alexander technique, 198
"All things come to those who
    wait," 289
Alpha waves, 196–197
Alternative approaches to quitting
    drinking, 222–229
Alternative programs (group),
    222–226
Alternative programs (individual),
    226–229
Amphetamines, 96
Anger, how to solve, 266
Antabuse, 221
Anxiety, how to solve, 265
Aromatherapy, 219–220
Assertiveness training, 181–184
Autogenic training/self-hypnosis,
    199
Avoiding drinking situations,
    257–258

Barbiturates, 95
Biofeedback, 196–197, 199
Blood sugar, 21, 25–26
Bodywork, 197
Borderline alcoholics, 28

Caffeine, 95, 160
Celebrations, enjoying without
    alcohol, 275
Cells
  adaptation to alcohol, 20, 29
  damage to, 31, 35–36
  functional failure, 31
  healthy cells, 36, 114–115
  rejuvenation of, 36, 121
Charity/altruism, 239–240
Checklists
  #1 Checklist of Medical
    Problems, 62–69
  #2 Alternatives to Drinking,
    106–112
  #3 Relaxers: What Works Best
    for You?, 181
  #4 22 Surefire Stress Reducers,
    185–189
  #5 Why I'm Not Drinking,
    260–263
  #6 Claim Your Prizes, 281–283
Chemical additives in food, 27, 159
Chemical deterrent to drinking,
    221
Chiropractic, 220–221
Cirrhosis, 57, 66
Clinics (a listing), 204–210
Cocaine (crack), 95
Codeine, 95
Constipation, how to solve,
    269–270
Contract to quit drinking, 250, 253
Convulsions, 20, 21
Cookbooks, 153–154
Coping with urges, 255–256
Counseling/psychotherapy,
    229–230
Cravings
  description of, 161–162

for addictive substances, 96
for alcohol, 26, 34, 116, 163
for food, 33–34, 116–117,
    162–163
for sugar, 25–27, 34, 161
how to cope with, 99–100, 105,
    161–164, 255–256

Decisions
  deciding to change, 52, 69–70,
    74–77, 98–99, 112–113,
    159–160, 250–253
  making effective decisions, 97,
    98, 112, 166, 264, 298–299
Deep rhythmic breathing, 177–179
Denial of problems, 37–44, 51
Depression, how to solve, 265–266
Detoxification
  as cause of death, 69
  in-patient care for, 69–70,
    204–210
  planning for, 69–70, 252
Diabetes, 28
Diarrhea, how to solve, 269–270
Diet
  absorption of nutrients, 143
  as way to cure disease, 35–36,
    114–116
  alcoholic diet, 33–35
  balanced for acid/alkaline,
    116–117, 119–121
  balanced for expansive/contrac-
    tive, 116–119
  diet options, 156, 159–160
  healthy diet, 36, 114–116,
    120–121, 156
  how to change to healthy diet,
    152–160
  recommended diet, 121–140
  when to cheat, 163–164
Dining out, 158–159
Disease
  alcoholism as a disease, 30, 34
  beliefs concerning disease, 30
  curing disease, 35–36, 39,
    114–115, 120–121, 192

definition, 30
disease process, 30–31, 34, 61–69
stopping the disease, 34, 35–36
Disturbed sleep, how to solve, 267
Disulfiram, 221
"Don't take anything too seriously," 290–291
"Do one thing at a time," 287–288
Drunkenness
   detox from, 69
   variables influencing, 13
DT's, 20, 21, 69, 270

Electron gun, 212
Eliminating the urge to drink, 121–140, 254–256
Endorphins, 161, 168, 169, 193
Enjoying yourself after quitting, 283–286
Evaluating your drinking
   benefits you get, 51–57
   problems caused by, 51–52, 57–74
   your decision to change, 51, 69, 74–77
"Everything changes," 290
Excuses for drinking, 39–41, 44–47
Excuses for not drinking, 259–263
Exercise
   aerobic (active), 169–173
   casual, 173–174
   weekly schedule, 171
Expressive arts therapy, 232–233

Family, how to solve problems with, 271–272
Fasting, 214–216
Feldenkrais method, 198
Fetal alcohol addiction, 24–25
Fetal Alcohol Syndrome, 24
Food
   beans, 122–123
   beverages, recommended, 135–136
   eggs, 131
   examples: acid/alkaline, 119–120

examples: expansive/contractive, 117–119
fish and fowl, 126–127
fruits, 128–129
milk and milk products, 129–130
natural sweeteners, 132
nightshade vegetables, 130–131
oils, 131–132
sea vegetables, 125
seasonings in cooking, 132–134
seeds and nuts, 125–126
table condiments, 134–135
vegetables, 123–125
what to avoid, 136–140
whole grains, 121–122
Food pyramid, 158
Four food groups system, 158
Freedom from alcohol
   breaking free, 300
   feeling free, 300–302
   staying free, 302–304
Friends, solving problems with, 273
Friendship, as way to inner strength, 189–191
Full-spectrum lighting, 231–232
Fuzzy thinking, how to solve, 271

Genetic inheritance, 23–24
Glutamine, 148–149
Goals
   seven steps to achieving, 299
   your important life goals, 295–298
Group therapy, 230–231
Growing in love, 240–241
Guilt, how to resolve, 267–268

Habits
   definition, 92, 93
   examples of, 93–95
   examples of addictions, 95–96
   how to break a habit, 96–102
   practice breaking habits, 102–104
Hallucinations, how to solve, 270
Having fun, 283–286

Healing with laughter, 211–212
Health
  alcohol's effects on, 57–74
  artificial feeling of, 30
  as inner strength, 166–167
  responsibility for, 5, 83, 84–85,
    152–160, 167, 192, 301
Healthful cooking
  various methods of preparation,
    140–141
  the best cookware, 142
Healthful eating
  chew well, 142–143
  don't eat before bedtime, 145
  don't overeat, 145–146
  eat only when hungry, 143–144
  relax when you eat, 144–145
  when you are hungry, eat, 144
"Hear the truth within," 292–293
Herbal remedies, 217–218
Heroin, 31, 95
Homeopathy, 220
How to be a winner, 298–299,
    302–303
Hug a friend, 233–234
Hypnosis, 198–199
Hypoglycemia, 32, 35
  healing hypoglycemia, 144
  hypoglycemic attack, 20, 25–27
  rate in alcoholic drinkers, 25

Inspirations
  definition, 287
  to make quitting easy, 287–294
Insulin, 25–26, 32
Internal healers, herbal, 218
International Association for
    Clear Thinking, 230–231
Intestinal cleansing, 216–217
Isoquinolines, 21, 31

Laxatives, 216
Life Process Program, 229
Light therapy, 231–232
Live-in programs (a listing), 204–210
"Live this very moment," 291

Loving relationships, as therapy,
    240–241
Lying, how to stop, 39–41

Make a contract to quit, 250, 253
Making your life a success, 295–
    299, 302–303
Malnutrition, 33
Marijuana, 96
Martial arts, various, 197
Massage
  acupressure/shiatsu, 195
  rolfing, 196
  sports, 196
  Swedish, 196
Mayo Clinic study
  validity of tests, 48
Medical check-up, 58, 61, 62, 70
Medical problems
  signs and symptoms, 62–66
  diagnosed, 66–69
Men for Sobriety, 223–224
Metabolism
  alcohol metabolism, 21–29
  "alcoholic metabolism," 22–30,
    31
  food metabolism, 31–32
  how to change metabolism,
    29–30, 32–33, 35
  hypoglycemic metabolism, 26
Minnesota Model, 205
Morphine, 31, 95

Neo-Reichian/bioenergetics, 198
Neuroelectric Therapy, 194–195
Nicotine, 95, 160
"No thanks, I don't drink," 259–
    260, 263
Nondrinking contract, specific sit-
    uation, 258

Ohashiatsu, 198
"Old endings are new beginnings,"
    289
Overeaters Anonymous, 27, 82
Overeating

cause of alcoholic metabolism,
    27–28
how to solve, 145–146, 268–269

"Patience is a virtue," 289
Personal notebook, 37
Picking a day to quit, 251–253
Polarity therapy, 198
Practices
    #1 Dialog with Body, 59–60
    #2 Try a Few Meetings, 84
    #3 Pick a Few Habits and Break
        Them, 102–104
    #4 Start Your New Diet, 165
    #5 Begin Doing It, 175
    #6 Assertive Responses: How to
        Remain Centered, 183–184
    #7 Find One Good Friend,
        190–191
    #8 Avoiding Drinking Situa-
        tions, 257–258
    #9 Three Ways to Keep Your
        Freedom, 303
Pregnancy, 24–25
Progressive relaxation, 179
Promise someone, 249
Protecting your drinking, 37, 38,
    39–40

Rational Behavioral Therapy,
    227–228
Rational-Emotive Therapy, 226
Rational Recovery, 206, 208,
    225–226, 230
Reasons for not drinking, 259–263
Reasons for quitting, 74–77
Relaxation techniques, 175–181
Religion, as healing, 234–235
Responsibility
    for health, 5, 83, 84–85,
        152–160, 167, 192, 301
    for freedom, 300–304
    for enjoying yourself, 283–286,
        290–291
Rewarding yourself, 280–283
Rubenfeld Synergy, 198

Save Our Selves, 224–225
Saving money, 276–277, 279–280
Saving time, 276–278
Secular Organizations for
    Sobriety, 224–225, 230
Sedatives, 95
Self reflection, 211
Setbacks, how to handle, 273–274
Sex
    as relaxation technique, 179–180
    how to solve problems with,
        272–273
Silymarin, 148
Sleep, how to solve problems
    with, 145, 267
Slips, how to avoid, 274
Social drinkers, 28
Solitude, as healing, 211
Spiritual healing
    a personal quest, 236
    the art of surrender, 239
    inspirations, 287–294
    many paths of yoga, 238
    meditation and meditative tech-
        niques, 236–237
    prayer, 237
    rebirthing, 238–239
Stress management/coping tech-
    niques, 185–189
Stress reducers, herbal, 217–218
Stretching/warm up exercises, 179
Subliminal suggestion, 202–204
Success rates
    AA, 1, 82, 205, 222
    acupuncture, 193
    affirmations, 204
    alternative recovery programs, 4,
        226, 227
    clinics and live-in programs,
        205, 206–209
    new alternatives, 4
    subliminal suggestion, 204
    visualization, 200, 204
Success with goals, 295–299
Supplements
    evaluation of, 146–147

Supplements *(cont)*
    guidelines for, 147–150
    three options, 150–152
Sugar addiction, 25–27, 34, 95,
    159–160, 161, 255

Tai Chi, 197
Tests for alcoholism
    Johns Hopkins Medical Institu-
        tion Test, 48–50
    NCADD test, 50
    One-question test, 38
Tolerance, 19, 20, 28
Trager mind-body integration, 198
Turn off your TV, 212–214
Twelve steps
    in AA, 81
    other twelve-step programs, 82

Unclear thinking, how to solve,
    271

Visions, 270
Visualization, 199–201, 204
Vitamin and mineral supplement,
    147–150
Vitamin C, 147–148, 149

When to quit, 251–253
Whole Person Approach to Recov-
    ery, 205, 206, 207, 208, 209,
    223
Withdrawal syndrome, 19–20, 24,
    26, 28, 34–35, 69–70
Women for Sobriety, 222–223, 230
Worksheets

#1 Denials and Excuses, 41–47
#2 Reasons for Drinking, 53–56
#3 Problems You'd Like to
    Avoid, 70–73
#4 Reasons for Quitting, 75–77
#5 My Decision about AA, 89–90
#6 Plan Your Own Exercise
    Program, 169–174
#7 Which Techniques Will You
    Do?, 241–243
#8 Your Master Plan, 248–249
#9 Contract to Quit Drinking,
    250–251
#10 Your Day, 253
#11 169 Ways to Cope with
    Urges, 256
#12 How Much Time Do You
    Save?, 277–278
#13 How Much Money Do You
    Save?, 279–280
#14 The Benefits of Not Drink-
    ing, 284–286
#15 Personal Life Goals, 296–298

Yoga, 176–177, 178, 181, 236, 238
You can change, 5, 96–97, 112–113,
    290, 303–304
"You can have this day for free,"
    293–294
"You can't have everything all at
    once," 292
Your evaluation of the program,
    305
"Your life is as long as you want
    it to be," 293

ABOUT THE AUTHOR

Jerry Dorsman developed his highly successful recovery program over a 14-year period. During this time he researched and tested hundreds of techniques to help with quitting drinking.

His original goal was to cure his own alcoholism. Dissatisfied with AA, the author pieced together a complete program and used it effectively when he quit drinking in 1981.

Since then, he has simplified this plan and improved it to reflect new discoveries in treatment and research. This resulted in an easy-to-follow yet all-inclusive approach. In its first edition, published in 1991, *How to Quit Drinking Without AA* became a top-selling recovery book; during the first two years it sold 23,000 copies. That edition was also translated into Spanish and released for distribution in fall 1993.

Jerry has appeared on more than 125 radio shows all over the United States and Canada and on two local TV shows. These shows represent a total audience numbering more than 9 million people. In addition, articles about his program and book reviews have appeared in *USA Today, The Philadelphia Inquirer, Your Health* magazine, *Better World* magazine, and almost every publication in the addiction and recovery field (including magazines, newsletters, and newsmagazines).

Jerry has also written various articles on recovery, published in *Professional Counselor* magazine, *Addiction & Recovery* magazine, *Journal of Rational Recovery, Northeast Recovery Networker,* and *Journey.*

He is an active member of NAADAC (National Association of Alcoholism and Drug Abuse Counselors) and he holds two degrees, one a high-honors degree in psychology. Jerry has worked as the director of a drug and alcohol counseling center in Pennsylvania, as a drug and alcohol counselor, as a mental health counselor, and as the director of numerous mental health programs in Maryland. Currently, he works for Upper Bay Counseling & Support Services, Inc., in Cecil County, Maryland, where, aside from administrative responsibilities, he provides group therapy for mental health clients who have problems with drug and alcohol addictions.